e-Communication Skills

A guide for primary care

Edited by

Louise Simpson
Paul Robinson
Mark Fletcher
Rob Wilson

Foreword by

Mike Pringle

Radcliffe Publishing
Oxford • Seattle

Radcliffe Publishing Ltd
18 Marcham Road
Abingdon
Oxon OX14 1AA
United Kingdom

www.radcliffe-oxford.com
Electronic catalogue and worldwide online ordering facility.

British Library Cataloguing in Publication Data

A catalogue record for this book is available from the British Library.

ISBN-10 1 85775 868 4
ISBN-13 978 1 85775 868 9

Typeset by Advance Typesetting Ltd, Oxford
Printed and bound by TJ International Ltd, Padstow, Cornwall

Language is only the instrument of science, and words are but the signs of ideas.

(Samuel Johnson)

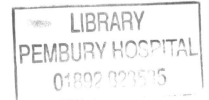

Contents

Frontispiece iii
Foreword ix
About the authors xi
About the contributors xii
Acknowledgements xiii
Dedications xiv

Part 1: Diagnosing the problem **1**
 1 About e-communication skills **3**
  Louise Simpson
   What could be different? 3
   Who is this book for? 5
   How to use this book 5
   References 5

 2 Introduction to e-communication skills **6**
  Louise Simpson
   The context: communications 6
   The context: informatics 7
   What patients say they want, and how informatics can help 8
   e-Communications: enabling shared decision-making 9
   e-Communications: enabling patient and clinician access to
    evidence-based guidance 9
   e-Communications: enabling interdisciplinary teamwork 10
   Barriers to e-communication 10
   Final thoughts 10
   References 11

 3 People communicate **12**
  Paul Robinson
   People communicate 12
   Models of communication 13

The nature of consciousness   15
Final thoughts   22
References   23

Part 2:   e-Communications in the clinical setting   **24**
4 e-Communication skills in the clinical setting   **26**
Paul Robinson
Setting the scene   26
Knowledge and expertise in the consultation   27
Using the computer in real consultations   33
Conclusion   34
References   34

5 Teams working e-together   **36**
Louise Simpson
Setting the e-scene   36
Starting at the beginning   37
Decision-making for e-teams   37
How teams make decisions   38
Interpersonal play versus task focus   38
Group e-think   39
Communication skills for e-teams   40
How teams might change   42
Issues for e-teams   43
A final thought   45
References   46

6 Information governance   **47**
Rob Wilson
What is information governance?   47
Why is information governance important?   49
What are the aims of information governance?   49
What are the requirements for primary care?   49
How can we *do* information governance in general practice?   50
What resources are available?   51
Final thoughts   51
References   52

7 Health inequalities and language diversity   **53**
Mark Gibson and Pam Turpin
Language diversity, health inequalities and patient
    information provision   53
How can technology help?   56
Conclusion   57
References   58

Part 3:   Practical matters   59
   8 Diagnosing the problem and finding a solution   61
      Mark Fletcher
         What is the problem?   61
         What is the likely solution?   62
         Making it happen   63
         A typical reputation audit   64

   9 Writing an e-communications strategy   65
      Mark Fletcher
         What is the starting point?   65
         What can we do about it?   66
         Outcomes   67
         Audiences   69
         Channels   74
         Messages   75
         Context   76
         Evaluation   77
         A final thought   77

  10 e-Communicating   79
      Mark Fletcher
         Electronic signatures   79
         The critical data   81
         Finding out what people think   82
         The header   83
         The body copy   84
         Developing an e-communications policy   87
         Reference   89

  11 The peculiarity of e-communication   90
      Mark Fletcher
         It's all on the record   90
         e-Games are entirely acceptable   90
         Managing e-risk   92
         Other ways of assessing communication risk   93

Part 4:   Resource pack   95
  12 Case study 1: People with sight loss, of South Asian origin,
      in Bradford   97
      Mark Gibson and Pam Turpin
         Introduction   97
         The evidence   98
         Discussion   100

13 Case study 2: The secondary care perspective　　**101**
Charlotte Bates
　Setting the scene　　101
　Communications requirements　　102
　Communication on an individual level　　103
　Interdepartmental communication　　103
　Communications: some problems and some solutions　　104
　Written communication　　106
　Telecommunications　　107
　Photocopying and facsimile　　108
　Computer systems and e-communication　　108
　Final thoughts　　109

14 Case study 3: Ditching the paper in Staffordshire　　**110**
Dai Evans
　Context　　110
　Development of e-working　　112
　Acquiring initial functional IT skills: a self-help group solution　　112
　Disseminating IT skills into the local community: local user
　　groups　　113
　Particular lessons in the development of electronic records　　113
　Organisational impacts on training: skinning the cat another
　　way　　114
　Some examples of personal change management　　115
　Process management in practice: an under-recognised
　　requirement　　116
　e-Working in the wider health community　　117
　Current position: computer-based records – successes
　　and holes　　120

15 Finding out more　　**122**
Louise Simpson
　Books, papers and journals　　122
　Web and CD-ROM resources　　122
　Organisations and their websites　　123
　Other materials: some useful addresses　　124

16 Glossary of abbreviations　　**125**

Index　　127

Foreword

Those of us who can remember the dramatic impact of the term 'evidence-based medicine' when it first entered our consciousness can see 'patient-centred care' becoming equally devalued by routine use. Yet both concepts continue to be fundamental drivers for the changes we are witnessing in clinical care and clinical communication.

Many of us share a vision in which the individual patient is an informed partner – the leading partner – in their care, and in which groups of patients support each other to use the skills of healthcare workers to the full. This requires public access to the information base of medicine, education in how to interpret and use it, and support in making rational choices.

Some fear that this will be the 'end of medicine'. It will certainly spell the death of paternalistic, closed medical decision-making, backed up by poor communication and an expectation of unthinking compliance. But, for most clinicians, this world will be liberating. Doctors, nurses and other healthcare professionals will be able to concentrate on ensuring that patients are as well-informed as they wish to be and are taking as much control over their health and illnesses as they can.

This revolution is, of course, driven by technology. Lay access to information previously only available to 'insiders', and to the uncertainties and controversies that surround it, will increase patients' knowledge of their conditions and their management. Access to medical records will help to contextualise that knowledge and allow each to monitor the effects of their healthcare choices. And new forms of communication will allow patients much greater access to the support of healthcare professionals.

There are significant inherent risks. Many people will continue to prefer to delegate healthcare decisions to 'professionals'; however, even these may want to seek second opinions more often.

Communication is a complex business and we are very familiar with the need to adjust our language in the light of verbal and non-verbal responses.

Electronic communication can never be a substitute for a consultation, just an augmentation that frees the consultation to address other important aspects of decision-making.

And we must recognise that the more information a person has, the greater is the scope for misunderstanding. Doctors use terms in agreed ways; patients may not understand their meaning in the same way. Health professionals are used to disagreement and uncertainty; the public often finds such lack of clarity unsettling. And, if we believe in personal informed choice, some choices made by patients may seem difficult to accept to health workers.

All these issues, and much more, are addressed in this excellent short guide to the new world of e-communication. As the technology surrounding healthcare becomes more all-pervasive, so the demands on health professionals will become more complex. The abilities to educate and support people in making choices will be highly prized. Above all, the ability to communicate in many media will be the hallmark of a skilled professional.

Professor Mike Pringle
National Clinical Lead for General Practice in
Connecting for Health
May 2005

About the authors

Louise Simpson has worked in and with the health scene since 1992, with experience as GP computer facilitator in Nottinghamshire, with the EMIS National User Group and SCHIN at the University of Newcastle. She currently works for the North East and North Cumbria clinical network for chronic fatigue syndrome and ME. Louise is author and co-editor of *e-Clinical Governance: a guide for primary care* (Radcliffe Medical Press, 2002) and she successfully achieved an MBA with a thesis entitled 'Organisational Learning in General Practice'.

Dr Paul Robinson is a GP in Scarborough. He also works in postgraduate medical education and is an Associate Director in Yorkshire Deanery. Paul's involvement in health informatics led him to work for the Sowerby Centre for Health Informatics for five years up to 2004. He is currently deputy chair of the RCGP health informatics standing group. Paul is author and co-editor of *e-Clinical Governance: a guide for primary care* (Radcliffe Medical Press, 2002).

Mark Fletcher is a partner with *reputation*, a strategic communications consultancy that works with many public sector organisations. He is author of *Managing Communication in Local Government* (Kogan Page, 1999).

Rob Wilson is lecturer in information systems management at the University of Newcastle upon Tyne. He is part of the FAME team at the Centre for Social and Business Informatics, which produced the generic framework for multi-agency working in health and social care. With ten years' experience of researching health informatics, Rob is widely published both nationally and internationally. He cites primary care prescribing informatics as a particular interest.

About the contributors

Charlotte Bates is a specialist registrar on the Northern Region A&E rotation, currently working in Newcastle General A&E.

Dai Evans is a GP working in the Peak District and a Clinical Advisor for PRIMIS at Nottingham University.

Mark Gibson is a sociolinguist and medical sociologist working as a research fellow at Leeds. He specialises in qualitative research in social and health sciences. His particular interests are clinician–patient communication and information about medicines.

Pam Turpin works for the Royal National Institute of the Blind (RNIB) and specialises particularly in quality of life and rehabilitation issues faced by older people with sight loss in the UK.

Acknowledgements

Thank you to the team at Radcliffe Publishing for your patience and encouragement. Also, thanks to Professor Mike Pringle, Charlotte Bates, Robin Beaumont, Dai Evans, Professor Michael Kidd, Mark Gibson, Steve O'Neill and Pam Turpin for your practical insights and your company along the way.

Louise's dedication
For Dr Alison Easton and Sandra Appleton – exceptional teachers
and communicators.

Paul's dedication
For Caz and Stex, Gate and Lu, Matt and Cat, My, Paul, Joan and Tommy.

Mark's dedication
For Hilary, Rachael, Roberta, Gregor and Ailis.

Rob's dedication
To my bright, shiny things – Lou, James and Alistair.

Part 1: Diagnosing the problem

About e-communication skills

Louise Simpson

What could be different?

There are always different ways to do things. The way we do things 'round here' might be how they have always been done, but new technologies, growing patient expectations and a changing society mean that they might not be the way we do things in the future. The banking system has changed, and, although it may not be fair to compare an essentially quantitative world with a vision for healthcare, there are lessons to be learned from this. Do I need to see the regional head of the bank to arrange a routine standing order? Do I have to arrange an appointment to see my bank statement, and pay a fee for the privilege? If I am truly responsible for my health – in the way I am responsible for my financial health – I need to be at the heart of the process. The *consultation* between the general practitioner and the patient is, for now, at the start, the middle and, often, at the end of things in healthcare, and even this represents a meaningful shift over the last 10 years, but there is further to go. The theme of trust will emerge again and again as we look at the way we do things round here – the way we communicate is through trust, the way information systems work for us needs trust, but, most of all, we need to trust patients to be at the centre of it all.

This book is about showing that communications are the responsibility of everyone in the primary care team; they are fundamental to patient care, practice administration, primary care trust management and population care. There is a range of resources and informatics available to enable primary care team members to enhance clinical and non-clinical communications, both internal (patients and practice) and external (primary care trust and the wider community).

The information age has changed the way we seek, consider and use data and knowledge, and has changed patterns of working and communicating. We can check our bank balance and do our shopping at any time on most days. The changes in healthcare are not just about access to information by people, patients, administrators, managers and clinicians, but also about the effect this has on interpersonal communications, decision-making and the wider business process.

Putting a computer on the desk in the consulting room – or taking a hand-held device to a 3 am call or assessment visit – not only allows the retrieval of important patient-centred information, but facilitates capture of the en-counter experience and fundamentally affects the dynamics of the interaction. Can we ever say 'just between ourselves' when there is a computer in the room? Well, of course we can, but the need for mindfulness when communi-cating is ever more important as we consider its impact on the whole healthcare experience and the most profound need for information governance.

With domestic e-mail and internet access booming, the way patients seek advice, guidance and reassurance is changing. The quality of its content is variable, yet the world wide web still offers an opportunity for primary care. Patients' expectations have altered – the computer is accepted as having its place in the care process – and still we must be attentive to the need for solid and sound information governance.

It has been reported that patients' satisfaction with the National Health Service (NHS) increased by 27% in the weeks following the NHS 50th birthday celebrations in 1998. The standards of care being experienced were consistent with other episodes in the NHS story, but the unified communi-cations campaign celebrating the unique role and place of the NHS was a single notable new factor.

The Association of Healthcare Communicators makes the following state-ment on its website (www.assochealth.org.uk):

> *The drive to strengthen communications across the NHS has never been more forceful as it sets about the task of delivering the targets set out in* The NHS Plan.[1] *As Nigel Crisp, NHS chief executive, said in* Shifting the Balance of Power:[2] *'Gone are the days when communications was a bolt-on activity. Now it is central to good management practice and crucial to building and maintaining public confidence in our health care system.'*

Increasing numbers of publications, policies and contract negotiations are making the link between quality healthcare and quality communications. What does this mean for primary care?

The guiding principles here are formative, developmental and reflective.

Who is this book for?

This book has been written with a number of people in mind. First, our focus is on the primary care consultation, the encounter between clinician and patient (the term 'patient' is used to describe the role of the citizen in the process). From there, we consider the context in which these encounters take place, and consider the communications needs and skills requirements for the wider primary care team: the administrative support and management specialists who all work towards that positive patient experience.

We also consider the opportunities and challenges offered by this e-world for healthcare communicators, recognising the contribution of this group in facilitating connection and well-being for the local population.

Lastly, we look through the window into the acute sector, and into the world of our local authority colleagues, and check out the real possibilities that modern informatics can offer, and try to signpost the pitfalls that might get in their way.

This book is a guide for primary care and covers the underpinning principles of communications, it also demonstrates how clinicians, managers and all members of the primary care team can exploit their informatics resources to enjoy and demonstrate excellence in communications.

How to use this book

This book has been written as an easy to use, dip in-and-out guide. It may be read from cover to cover, or you may choose to pick out one section and use that first. As well as being a guide to support individual knowledge development about both informatics and communications in primary care, it can also be used as a teaching resource, either as background reading or by using sections to prompt small group work.

References

1   Department of Health (2000) *The NHS Plan*. Department of Health, London. www.dh.gov.uk/assetRoot/04/05/57/83/04055783.pdf
2   Department of Health (2002) *Shifting the Balance of Power: the next steps*. Department of Health, London. www.dh.gov.uk/assetRoot/04/05/35/54/04073554.pdf

2

Introduction to e-communication skills

Louise Simpson

The context: communications

No one in primary care works in isolation. Communication is a foundation stone on which the clinician–patient relationship is based in primary care, and it is at the heart of the modernising NHS.

Good communication requires engagement, promotion, time and as much listening as speaking. Done well, it positively transforms both the clinician's and the patient's experience. Communication seems like an easy thing to do, yet it often heads any list of frustrations and complaints. So, with many millions of pounds being invested in the NHS information technology (IT) infrastructure, and accompanying service improvement, is a new communications paradigm emerging? What are the implications for those of us who work with patients? Will we need a new set of communications skills?

In 2003, the British Medical Association (BMA) published a consultation document *Communication Skills Education for Doctors: a discussion paper*, which stated that:

> *Good communication skills are recognised by the medical and other healthcare professions as central elements in demonstrating appropriate attitudes and professional development. The benefits of effective communication include good working relationships, increased patient satisfaction and improved health for patients. Undoubtedly, there are barriers to*

effective communication ranging from personal attitudes to the limitations placed on doctors by the organisational structures in which they work.[1]

The BMA rightly cites the artificial construct of the organisation as a potential barrier. But organisational boundaries will be overturned in the future. With the NHS Care Records Service, the vision of the patient-centred information record comes a step closer. The motto is 'right information, right time, regardless of location'. Appropriate access to information, 24 hours a day, is the aim. A central data 'spine' will enable information-sharing across agencies, organisational structures, teams and professions.

With so much being spent on IT support for the care process, pausing for a moment to reflect on how to build on existing communications skills seems timely. The computer is as common as the stethoscope on the clinical desktop, but the new models found in 'Connecting for Health' (formerly the National Programme for IT (NPfIT), a means of driving forwards the implementation of modern information systems and technology across the NHS)[2] will change the experience of using electronic health records for good. And if one of the barriers to good communications is conflicting advice, how can we manage in a world of information overload?

Combining the drive to computerise with recognition of the importance of quality communications is the starting point for this book. Quality communications – clinical, organisational and external – are the responsibility of everyone in the general practice team, and this book looks at what informatics resources are available to help to improve them and, therefore, the quality of patient care in the modernising NHS.

The context: informatics

'Connecting for Health' is changing the way healthcare computing is designed, built and operated. Five clusters structure management and implementation, and new communities and alliances are emerging as a result. The technical infrastructure is getting a mighty boost and the IT architectures that have dominated the NHS for over a decade are being replaced with a new technical model, the result of the largest procurement of IT systems ever undertaken. The NHS Care Records Service is just that – the NHS now buys a service, not systems.

The document, *Delivering 21st Century IT for the NHS*,[3] was published in June 2002 and its aims were to connect the delivery of *The NHS Plan*[4] with the capabilities of modern technologies, to:

- support the patient and the delivery of services designed around the patient, quickly, conveniently and seamlessly

- support staff in the delivery of integrated care, through effective electronic communications, better learning and knowledge management, cut the time to find essential information (notes, test results) and make specialised expertise more accessible
- improve the management and delivery of services by providing good quality data to support national service frameworks, clinical audit, governance and management information.

The key principle is that care services are designed around the needs of patients and service users, they are not based on NHS institutions.

The core of the strategy is to take greater control over specification, procurement, resource management, performance management and delivery of the information and IT agenda.

In August 2002, the specification for an integrated care records service (now the 'NHS Care Records Service') was published by the Department of Health. This outlined proposals for a life-long electronic health records service, providing information support to care processes whether they took place in the primary, community, secondary, tertiary or mental health sectors. For clinicians, this means having the right information at the right time. It means no longer seeing patients without knowing what has happened to them, and where. It means no longer finding fragments of the story in multiple paper records. It means the patient's story being one story – one patient working with many people from different teams, in many places: like healthcare works, really.

What patients say they want, and how informatics can help

A report by the Lothian University Hospitals NHS Trust explored patients' views on communications (as reported in the Scottish Executive's report, *Talking Matters*):[5]

- 60% complained about a lack of involvement in decisions about their care
- 60% said they were given no information about resuming normal activities after treatment
- 46% said they were given inaccurate information about how they would feel after treatment
- 33% said they had been given no explanation of test results
- 23% complained of nurses and doctors saying different things.

Although this is an extremely brief summary of the report's findings, a number of communications themes emerge:

- the need for shared decision-making
- the need to access and share evidence-based clinical guidance
- the need for interdisciplinary and multidisciplinary teamwork.

The informatics domain offers a number of solutions to these three themes and we will explore each of them now. However, a peek at the final section of this book will reveal a range of other resources, approaches and ideas. But, back to our snapshot of solutions.

e-Communications: enabling shared decision-making

Imagine the computer as a resource to support the patient and the clinician in the consultation encounter. It provides a prompt, a source of knowledge and a place to record the experience of that encounter. But it is also an artefact in itself. The computer can act as a third party – 'Look what it says here' – is a technique that facilitates discussion and helps patients to consider and review a piece of knowledge or proposed action without a sense of challenging the doctor, or of confrontation. The computer as 'honest broker' or third-party facilitator is a theme that runs throughout e-communication and enables shared decision-making. This is why patients will bring the actual computer printouts from their internet searches to the surgery with them – using an external artefact not only acts as an aide-memoire but also gives patients a degree of confidence to discuss the contents in a non-challenging way.

e-Communications: enabling patient and clinician access to evidence-based guidance

Knowledge changes all the time, and the rate of journal publication – one source and type of evidence – is a speeding colossus in its own right. It is impossible to keep up to date with all the latest guidance, research or evidence for every condition that presents in primary care. Computers are good at finding things and displaying them quickly, without the need for masses of paper and filing. Use the computer to support access to evidence – patients do.

e-Communications: enabling interdisciplinary teamwork

Professor Michael Kidd writes, 'As a general practitioner I believe that my patients are most at risk when they cross the boundaries in our healthcare system.'[6] The paper medical record is a well-established communications tool. A glance at a paper record enables clinicians to see why a patient last presented, the key summary facts about that patient and a snapshot of encounters with colleagues in the acute sector or in the wider practice team. If you can sift your way through it.

Computer software can be a good way of organising information, patient-based information, better than paper can. With the developments in the NHS Care Records Service, and the emergence of a data 'spine', the ability to view quickly the key events in a person's health story is an attractive opportunity. The key events will be available to the appropriate healthcare professional, regardless of geographic or organisational restrictions, within hours. Medications prescribed in hospital will be entered on the data spine, which is then available electronically to the team in primary care, with appropriate confidentiality considerations. Communications between disciplines in the same team and between teams working in different care settings is helped by informatics.

Barriers to e-communication

It is an old chestnut, but 'rubbish in, rubbish out' is a crucial point for the e-communications paradigm. Information governance offers a framework for information quality, for confidentiality and security – important themes for informatics and communications. It is essential to be able to trust data on which decisions might be made. If data have been entered by an anonymous person from a large care provider in another part of the county, or country, clinicians in the primary care setting need a framework by which trust can be engendered. It is too early to seek an information governance 'kitemark', but understanding the principles of information governance is one way of engendering trust.

Final thoughts

Will we need a new set of communications skills to deal with the fast-paced developments in IT? Maybe a complementary set of tools to our communications toolkit is one way of looking at this dilemma. Patients do not want clinicians to spend the valuable seven-and-a-bit minutes of their consultation in typing or following a mouse about the screen: but that does not preclude a middle way, whereby access to knowledge – both in terms of evidence-based guidance and the patient's story – is enabled by the technical infrastructure.

Beyond the consultation, organisational learning and wider population communications can be facilitated by the opportunities offered by new technology and the new national programme drivers. But, of course, trust is of paramount importance in the realms of communications and informatics, information governance provides both a framework for trust and a foundation for e-communications.

References

1   British Medical Association (2003) *Communication Skills for Doctors: a discussion paper*. BMA, London.
2   Department of Health (2000) *Connecting for Health*. Department of Health, London.
3   Department of Health (2002) *Delivering 21st Century Support for the NHS*. Department of Health, London.
4   Department of Health (2000) *The NHS Plan*. Department of Health, London. www.dh.gov.uk/assetRoot/04/05/57/83/04055783.pdf
5   Scottish Executive (2003) *Talking Matters: developing the communication skills of doctors*. Scottish Executive, Edinburgh.
6   Kidd M (2001) Personal communication.

3

People communicate

Paul Robinson

She wears an Egyptian ring, it sparkles before she speaks.
(Bob Dylan, 'She Belongs to Me')

Communication and the communications industries dominate modern life. New technologies of mobile communication enable people to stay in touch with one another across any distance and throughout the day and the working week. Good communication skills are regarded as essential competencies for many jobs, including medicine and nursing.

In this chapter we set the context by looking at communication in general terms. In doing this we will go beyond traditional models of communication, applying new understandings of how the brain and the mind work. These insights from complexity theory, neuroscience and social learning in communities will inform our journey through the world of e-communication in healthcare.

People communicate

People communicate. All the time, from before birth until death, awake and asleep. In some ways verbal communication dominates, whether written or spoken. Examples are talking and listening, reading and writing, broadcasting and viewing. As well as these *inter*personal examples we have *intra*personal communication, which includes the 'inner voice' through which we talk to ourselves.

Of course, we also communicate with non-verbal sounds, such as music, through vision and image, through touch and smell. We can communicate factual information, abstract concepts, ideas and emotions.

In some ways this range of communication seems to define the human species and set us apart from other animals. This is one of the fascinations of looking at early cave art: maybe we are looking at a point of demarcation between human and pre-human?

Probably not. The work Darwin began when he started to challenge the supposed boundary between humans and other animals remains unfinished. All our ways of communicating have evolved from ways used by other mammals and other genera. This evolution has largely been additive: this means that much of the way we communicate is shared with other species. Desmond Morris pointed this out in his books *Man Watching* and *The Naked Ape*.[1,2] It is there to be seen in television nature series such as David Attenborough's *Life of Mammals*. Darwin himself got there first in 1872 with his book *The Expression of Emotions in Man and Animals*.[3] Even language, which is held by many to be a definingly human characteristic, is based on communication through symbols: a characteristic that is found across the animal kingdom. Of course, the way that humans have picked up the ball of communication by symbol and run with it is unique. Language seems to dominate communication but, as we shall see later in this chapter, this dominance is illusory. When people communicate they do so as mammals in the first instance, they communicate as people second.

Models of communication

One of the leading contributions to consultation skills teaching in recent years has come from the work of Kurtz, Silverman and Draper. Their two books draw from a composite model.[4] This model is itself a composite of three standard models of communication, described below.

Shannon

This is an informatics model (Figure 3.1) that was developed to support analysis of telephone systems. Its main features are that:

- the language in which information is carried down the channel is not the same as the representation of that information at either source or destination
- distortion may occur at encoding or decoding and along the channel.

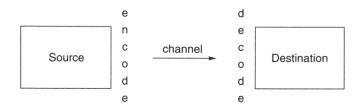

Figure 3.1 Information theory model (Shannon).

With interpersonal communication there are three channels: the verbal; the vocal (tone, timbre and volume); and the non-verbal (body language). The potential distortions at the encoding and decoding phases are legion and include affective, contextual and experiential. In addition, the three channels carry a lot more information than an individual recipient can be aware of; affective and other personal factors will determine which parts of the message are attended to.

Baker

This is a psychological model.[5] It starts from the premise that the purpose of communication is to achieve silence, not more communication. The outcome of communication is expressed as to how much 'psychic tension' is present in the silence, that is, how comfortable it is.

Baker correlated the comfort of the silence to the degree to which the two participants identify with each other. The more complete the reciprocal identification, the more effective the communication. This goes some way to explain why pharmaceutical representatives and other salesmen keep records of their clients' interests and always engage in conversation around these topics before moving on to business.

Dance

Dance's model is a simple helix (see Figure 3.2).[6]

The point of this is that each interaction in a communication affects each of the participants, and so has an effect on what follows. Each exchange of dialogue is built on the previous one: this places great emphasis on how conversations open.

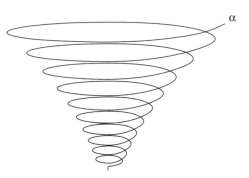

Figure 3.2 Dance's model.

A summary of principles

There are several basic principles of communication that follow from these models:

- all communication, even the simplest information-giving is interactive
- the aim of communication is to achieve shared understanding
- to do this you have to know what the recipient knows (or what his or her models are) before you start
- the message received is not the same as the message sent
- because of this it is necessary to check out what the recipient thinks your message was.

Further information on these models can be found at www.swaysides. demon.co.uk/commods.html.

The nature of consciousness

These models form the basis of much of our current understanding of communication, and the way that they have been applied to medical communication skills by Riccardi and Kurtz underlines this.[4] Their skill set for the medical consultation can be applied to teaching in various settings. In the setting of developing teaching and consulting skills the models make sense and fit with people's common-sense view of what is happening when they communicate with other people.

This means that when I am in conversation with someone, it feels as if I listen to what they say and make a reasoned response. It also feels as if I can monitor the conversation, plan the direction it will take, notice things about how the other person sounds and appears: I use this information to direct events and plan them. This is part of a more general feeling that my conscious awareness (by which I mean the part of me that sees and hears, that plans and thinks as my inner voice) resides in my head: somewhere behind my eyes. This idea underlines Descartes' famous attribution to the pineal of being the seat of the soul: which he thought of as being completely different in nature from the body. This notion, which Dennett calls 'Cartesian theatre',[7] is widespread. It seems now to be illusory on several counts, as we will discover.

The first illusion is that there is one single site for consciousness. New methods of brain imaging allow researchers to locate activity in the conscious brain very accurately in both time and site. What has emerged from this has overturned many of the suppositions of neurology. There is no single site for consciousness, which appears to be an emergent property of the whole brain. The new imaging techniques show that many diverse parts of the brain are involved in the perception of a visual image. These go far beyond what were previously classified as the primary and secondary visual cortices. Perception of vision involves a huge amount of pre-afferent activity: the traffic from cortex towards the retina being about ten times as heavy as from retina to cortex. Other perceptions, such as pain, are even more heavily represented in what used to be referred to as 'motor pathways'.

The second major finding from this work is that it takes time for us to be consciously aware of seeing something. The time delay is typically just less than 0.5 seconds. Changes in brain activity occur progressively from the instant that a visual stimulus is presented, but the subject is not consciously aware of seeing it for half a second. This lends weight to the notion of consciousness being constructed from activity in the neural network that makes up the brain. Another consequence of this line of thought is that what we are conscious of seeing when we look at something is not the thing itself, but our constructed simulation of it.

The third illusion is that when we are, for instance, playing a ball sport such as tennis we watch the ball and decide (in the bit of 'me' behind my eyes) how to hit the ball back. Professional tennis players hit the ball so fast in the service that it only takes 0.3 seconds to travel from racket to other end of the court. Yet the receiving player often not only gets a racket to the ball, but often makes a purposeful shot: sometimes a winner. Either top sportsmen are very good at guessing what their opponents are going to do, or there is some other way that they are able to see the ball and react appropriately to it.

Domasio[8] describes a route that links the optic pathway, via the superior colliculi on the thalamus to basal ganglia, which control movement. This, evolutionarily older, pathway has a latency of 0.2–0.3 seconds. Furthermore, practised responses to a stimulus (for example, pressing the car brake pedal in response to a red traffic light) have a latency of 0.1–0.2 seconds. This, by the way, is the rationale behind the way that false starts are detected in athletics. Any movement on the starting blocks that occurs within 0.1 second of the gun being fired is counted as a false start, on the grounds that it must have been initiated before the gun was fired.

So the body can respond quickly to stimuli and, after training, this response can be purposeful. The point is, though, that the response occurs before the individual has consciously seen the stimulus. The response does not rely on the cerebral cortex. This is one reason why sportsmen are often unable to give a coherent account of play until they have seen the video. On this timescale our symbol-based rational consciousness is always a few hundred milliseconds behind the action. Consciousness is a post hoc rationalisation or narrative: the feeling of what happens, the remembered present.

Simulation in the brain

Domasio's view of consciousness is that it arises from images, or simulations, of the body's internal state, which is directly linked to emotions, and of the external environment.[8] In developing this idea he talks about emotion as arising from attraction or repulsion: in evolutionary terms the way single cell organisms will move towards food and away from the noxious. This places emotion as a movement or a reaction, and Domasio suggests that the way that the brain 'images' sensory inputs is in terms of the body's response to them. The body's response to a stimulus or an agent feeds into the simulation that we construct of it. In child development, this is an explanation of the importance of handling objects in creating the link between patterns of light and objects.

In addition we simulate social relationships and culture. The cerebral cortex is hugely complex in its interconnections and this neural network is an ideal medium for supporting such a simulation. This capacity for simulation and memory is almost boundless. This scope is in sharp contrast to working memory.

Working memory in humans is quite limited: it can only hold between seven and nine items. If they are not allowed time to rehearse and repeat the numbers, people can only recall seven to nine random digits. Similarly, if someone is asked to match four items to four colours, and there is no connecting pattern, they are unable to do it if they are only able to use working memory. This does not mean that our working memory is 'eight-bit', in computer terms. What we can hold on to are not digits, but concepts or symbols, or episodes of a story. One of the ways that we deal with the small size of our working memory is to use story or narrative to structure memory. People who do memory tricks do so by placing apparently disconnected facts in a story, or on features of a repeating visual image (such as the arches in a cathedral nave), thus linking them in a way that allows them to be retrieved. The other way is by using single words to carry more and more sophisticated meanings. The effect of this is that, provided the meanings are shared, communication can be concise and economical. For instance a telephone number such as 72863624 may not be easy to recall as a string of digits. Much easier to think of it as 72 86 36 24 (as the French would). Recollection is easier still if you have local knowledge and recognise 72 as an area code, and 86 as the code for a single exchange; if you have a mathematical mind and see a connection between 36 (12×3) and 24 (12×2). We make up for the small capacity of working memory by adding patterns and stories. This takes time, but we have near limitless capacity for working with story. In the instant, though, all we have are the eight slots.

Working memory is equivalent to conscious attention: the 'I' behind my eyes. As Figure 3.3 shows, this is generated from the simulation of the world that is produced by the cortex. This diagram is reminiscent of Plato's cave (Figure 3.4). Because of the mismatch between the capacity of the cortex and the working memory, we are consciously aware of only part of what is contributing to the simulation that produces consciousness.

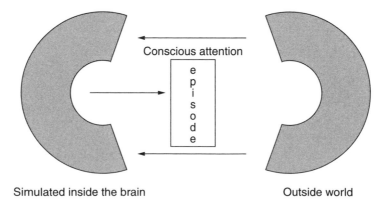

Simulated inside the brain   Outside world

Figure 3.3 Simulation in the brain.

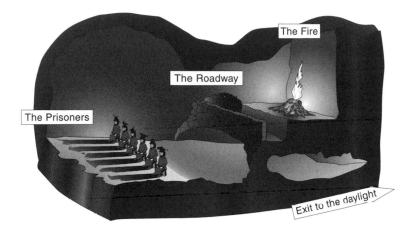

Figure 3.4 Plato's cave.

The prisoners think that what they are looking at is the real world. In fact, it is a projection of shadow's cast by puppets that are on the roadway and backlit by the fire. Daylight and the rest of the world is beyond the cave.

What has this to do with our understanding of communication?

Narrative and story

Inventions such as writing, printing and now word-processing on computers have all reduced our reliance on the oral tradition of story-telling. Few people can perform epics of story-telling that take hours or days, although the tradition does persist outside the developed world. Even so, much of our conversation, and much of the speech that takes place in a medical consultation, is in the form of stories. I think that our reliance on stories stems from the mismatch between the almost infinite capacity of the cerebral cortex and the eight-slot working memory that is our conscious attention.

Stories are made up of episodes. The archetypal episode is:

- it was like this
- then that happened
- now it is like *this*.

Thus an episode takes up three slots. Working memory is just big enough to contain two episodes and the link between them at the same time. Story is the reading-off of single episodes: sense is made through the thread of narrative that links up these subunits. When people are retelling long stories they do not recite them verbatim, they retain the narrative thread and major landmarks in the story, but improvise much of the language used.

Although story is sequential, and in that sense linear, the structure can be elaborated. As in some children's stories, the narrative can be recursive and repetitive. Story allows complicated ideas to be expressed in a way that our limited working memories can cope with.

Social factors and meaning

The other way that complicated concepts can be transmitted through language (a limited set of verbal symbols) is by using a particular word as shorthand for a concept: for instance think of the meaning that lies behind medical terms such as *hypertension* or *functional*. One way to describe this process is to call it *jargon*. Understanding of the terms is restricted to an in-group who have had the experience and training that lets them share the meaning.

Of course this is frustrating to people who are not members of the in-group, but establishing shared sense-making of terms and language is an essential aspect of people working in groups. Etienne Wenger explores this in his book *Communities of Practice*.[9] This book makes the point that all meanings of terms are socially determined. Once we are immured in a jargon it becomes hard to discuss the topic without using words in their specialised sense. It may be difficult to do, but the skill of expressing technical ideas in everyday language is essential for those of us who talk to patients.

Subliminal inputs get into the simulation

I have made the point in Figure 3.3 that information can influence the cerebral cortex without passing through conscious attention. My hunch is that much more gets into our heads this way than any other. Of course this is difficult to prove, but it is the only way that I can explain two things that I have experienced when working with videotapes of consultations or teaching sessions. One of these is the way that everyone in the group seems to see something different when looking at the video-recording. Everyone has a different (partial) experience. This is not surprising when you think about the amount of information that is presented on a video screen.

The other thing that comes out of watching these videos is that you can see the power of non-verbal communication. The demeanour and mood of one person on the screen is affected directly by the other person in the consultation. Often, when the players in the original consultation are in the watching group they are not aware of this transfer until it is pointed out to them.

It has been estimated that about 90% of interpersonal communication is through the non-verbal channel. Again it is difficult to confirm this, but it does serve to emphasise that the cognitive and verbal aspects (of which humanity is so proud) are only a small part of what goes on.

To an extent it is factual information that is conveyed verbally, and emotions and feelings that are displayed by posture and facial expression. Experienced practitioners, of medicine and of teaching, become very adept at recognising occasions where there is conflict between verbal and non-verbal messages. These are significant moments, characterised by a pattern of behaviour. A large part of expertise in any field is down to pattern recognition: patterns become so familiar that they are acted on without conscious thought.

Most well-rehearsed responses become automatic

Think back to the time when you were learning to drive a car. Every action of the beginner learner-driver is deliberate. You do not just change gear, you have to remember to press the clutch ('Which pedal is that?') grope for the gear stick ('Which gear am I in?' 'Which one do I want to go to?' 'Which movement does that need?'). Meanwhile the car continues to move forwards, the tension in the arm that is still holding the steering wheel has moved the car towards the middle of the road: when your attention returns to the road you are in a different place. As an expert driver a gear-change becomes just part of a manoeuvre, such as overtaking a lorry, that you perform with no more thought than you would give to walking along a pavement. In fact, sometimes after a journey along a familiar road you will have no recollection of driving the car at all. The whole thing has happened (perfectly safely) while you were thinking about something else altogether and you let your body (and eyes) get on with the job 'on their own'. This is because you are an expert driver.

It is the same with expert sportsmen, like tennis players. After spending many hours in rehearsing a particular shot, say, a forehand drive down the line, the shot becomes an automatic response. Not only that; the pattern of a ball that has the right flight to be hit in that way becomes automatically recognised. After this level of rehearsal play becomes automatic: being 'in the zone' means being stimulated enough to work hard, but relaxed enough to let the body and brain get on with playing tennis. Too much pressure and the player starts worrying about the detail of what they are doing and performance drops off.

Only a few people have that level of expertise at sport. We are all experts at communication: we have been practising for hours each day from before birth. Consequently, our actions are often like those of the tennis player or expert driver. That is, we recognise patterns and produce appropriate responses automatically. Literally, we do things and say things without thinking about them. For example, an expert consulter who sees someone looking depressed or upset will make an empathic remark, or use silence, without thought.

Final thoughts

Earlier in this chapter I wrote this passage:

> ... when I am in conversation with someone, it feels as if I listen to what they say and make a reasoned response. It also feels as if I can monitor the conversation, plan the direction it will take, notice things about how the other person sounds and appears: I use this information to direct events and plan them. This is part of a more general feeling that my conscious awareness (by which I mean the part of me that sees and hears, that plans and thinks as my inner voice) resides in my head: somewhere behind my eyes.

That is very much the feeling that I have when writing this: before I type I am saying the words to an imaginary audience, sometimes to one of my co-authors. The sense of my arguments in this chapter is that this feeling is an illusion, though it may be a necessary illusion.

We are mammals. Although we have developed a superstructure of linguistic communication, which is amazingly rich and productive, this is based on a system of non-verbal communication that is close to our emotional state and works faster than thought. The totality of what we communicate is more than what we intend.

This book is about e-communication. Most traffic in the electronic world is text. So do different rules apply? Can we forget about this mammalian emotional subliminal stuff? Well, not really. Stories about online romances are familiar enough. The whole thing of 'netiquette' has been constructed to try to avoid emotional problems in online communication. Who has not been 'flamed' on an e-mail discussion list? I am sure that you are astute enough to have noticed what I wrote two paragraphs earlier, comparing the task of typing to talking to people in the room. It is this relation between text_on_screen and the social and emotional worlds that underpins this book.

We will return to this theme.

References

1   Morris D (1978) *Man Watching: Field guide to human behaviour.* Triad, London.
2   Morris D (1994) *The Naked Ape: A zoologist's study of the human animal.* Vintage, London.
3   Darwin C (1999) *The Expression of Emotions in Man and Animals.* Definitive edition. Fontana Press, London.
4   Riccardi VM and Kurtz SM (1983) *Communication and Counselling in Health Care.* Charles C Thomas, Springfield, IL.
5   Baker SI (1955) The theory of silences. *Journal of General Psychology* **53**: 159.
6   Dance FEX (1967) Toward a theory of human communication. In: Dance FEX (ed.), *Human Communication Theory.* Holt, Reinhart & Winston, New York.
7   Dennett DC (1996) *Darwin's Dangerous Idea: Evolution and the meanings of life.* Penguin Science, London.
8   Domasio A (1999) *The Feeling of What Happens: Body and emotion in the making of consciousness.* Harcourt Brace & Co., New York.
9   Wenger E (1999) *Communities of Practice: learning, meaning and identity.* Cambridge University Press, Cambridge.

Part 2:
e-Communications
in the clinical setting

4

e-Communication skills in the clinical setting

Paul Robinson

This chapter describes the knowledge flows in the consultation and the impact that a computer can have on a consultation. Some research into computer use in general practice is reviewed, and we look at practical aspects of how to use a computer during a consultation without damaging rapport with the patient. Ways in which these practical skills can be used in everyday consultations are also discussed.

Setting the scene

Computers are now commonplace in consulting rooms in primary care; they are as much a part of the desk furniture as the stethoscope and ophthalmoscope. Although some practices make full use of the computer's potential to support electronic records and clinical governance, others only use a computer as an administrative tool and to issue prescriptions.

In the UK it is government policy that electronic records and electronic transfer of information become the norm, and the appropriate use of information technology (IT) is an essential part of the drive to improve quality in the NHS.

Knowledge and expertise in the consultation

A model of knowledge use

In a project looking at use of knowledge in general practitioner consultations, Robinson and Heywood[1] evolved the model summarised in Figure 4.1.

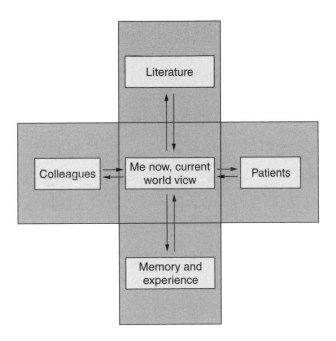

Figure 4.1 Knowledge use in the consultation.

In this research, as many as 170 knowledge items could be identified in a 10-minute consultation. The knowledge used in the consultation could be mapped out according to the four categories outlined in Figure 4.1, with practitioners accessing knowledge from different sources in turn.

Table 4.1 shows how, in a routine consultation, the general practitioner (GP) is using knowledge gained from different sources. All this information is available in the consultation, either from the patient or from the GP's memory. This is the traditional view of the expert–client relationship: the expert acquires knowledge through initial training, experience and continual professional development, and then dispenses this knowledge to the client.

Table 4.1 Knowledge flow in part of a consultation for cystitis

Patient	Memory/experience	Colleagues	Literature
This woman has blood in her urine, and it burns when she passes urine			
			These are the symptoms of cystitis, which is common
			Blood in urine can indicate serious conditions
She had a similar episode last year, which settled with antibiotics			
	Some people are very worried when they see blood in their urine		
She does not look worried			
			Nitrites in the urine strongly suggests infection
She has ++ nitrites			
		We normally check MSU in every suspected case of urine infection	
			A three-day course of trimethoprim is usually sufficient treatment for cystitis
		Practice policy is to use a five-day course of trimethoprim	
	I can remember failure of treatment with a three-day course		

MSU = mid-stream urine.

Most of the time the expert's knowledge and experience are sufficient. If not, the four different sources of knowledge can be consulted: the GP can ask a colleague (either another GP or a specialist); go to textbooks or journals; or look at the notes of another patient with a similar problem. Expertise is deployed in the choice of knowledge source, and the way in which it is accessed and then interpreted.

The desktop computer fundamentally alters the expert–client relationship. All the different knowledge sources are potentially available through the electronic record, local and networked information sources. PRODIGY is one example of an electronic knowledge source (although it is fundamentally different to electronic textbooks and local protocols as it actively, rather than passively, offers this information to you). Now that complex clinical questions can be answered in seconds, and guidance through PRODIGY is available instantly, the transaction changes from: 'What can I tell you about ...?' to 'What can we find out about ...?'

How computer use affects the consultation

The literature focuses on two aspects of computer use in the consultation. The first relates to perceptions of how a computer affects the dynamics of the consultation. Medical students are taught the skills of history-taking, examination, ordering investigations and giving treatment as if these were separate elements. At some point in their clinical training doctors learn to run these skills together and do them simultaneously at the bedside, retiring to the nurses' station to write up their notes. Colin Douglas describes this in his book *The Houseman's Tale*.[2] Most GPs cling to this habit, no doubt encouraged by the emphasis on the doctor–patient relationship in consultation skills training. This results in the computer simply being used to record information at the end of the consultation. Concerns about losing rapport with patients when using the computer in the consultation were voiced by GPs in the evaluation of Phase 2 of PRODIGY.[3] Als[4] found many of the patients she interviewed in Denmark were uncertain what their GP was doing when he or she was using the computer.

The other aspect noted in the literature is the observed effects of computer use. Most of this work is a few years old now and the computer use studied was related to the generation of prescriptions. This work has shown that when the computer is used:

- the doctor spends more time looking at screen than at paper[5]
- the doctor reduces the time spent interacting with the patient[6]
- there is increased length of consultation[7]

- there is increased doctor-initiated, as opposed to patient-initiated, content of the consultation
- there is increased medical compared to social content of the consultation.

Greatbach *et al.*,[8] looked at communication skills and found that using a computer does interfere with doctors' communication behaviour, but this interference could be minimised by practice and experience (allowing 'backgrounding' of use of the computer).

The limitation of this work is that, until now, it has looked at a relatively mechanical part of the consultation: the generation of prescriptions. One implication of information or decision support in the consultation is that it requires the practitioner's full attention and cannot be backgrounded. Another implication is that the practitioner is required to engage with the computer during the main body of the consultation so that computer use cannot be left until it ends.

The iiCR project and a skills-based approach

The Information in the Consulting Room (iiCR) project looked at the triadic consultation (general practitioner–patient–computer) from the communication skills point of view. A group at the Sowerby Centre analysed videotapes of consultations submitted by GPs who were comfortable with computer use in the consultation. From this material a series of communication skills were identified and classified, and these can be used to enable practitioners to use computers in the consultation without damaging rapport with their patients. In fact, use of these skills can *enhance* rapport. A training package to disseminate these skills was then developed.

From videotapes and training sessions it was found that it is possible to use a computer during the course of the consultation and maintain rapport with the patient. However, it is not possible to do both at the same time. If your attention is fully engaged with the computer it is not possible to listen to the patient, understand what they are saying and respond appropriately. This is because multitasking relies on backgrounding some or all of the tasks that you are engaged in. Talking and listening to the patient can take your full attention, as can the computer if you are having to read, understand and base your decisions on the information offered by it. The trick is to avoid trying to do both things at once, by either directing the consultation or making use of the structure of the consultation.

When the doctor's attention is on the computer screen there is likely to be a pause in the conversation, and patients often say important things after pauses in the conversation. One of the risks of using the computer, therefore, is that the patient will say something important while your attention is directed at the screen, and you may miss important cues or the 'While I'm here doctor ...' offering, which is often the true reason for attending. As previously mentioned, Als[4] found that the patient may be uncertain about what the doctor is doing when using the computer. It is therefore possible that the patient may assume that you are listening when you are not.

Practical tips

There are several different ways to cope with these problems. None are better than others – different ways suit different practitioners at different times. They should be regarded as different tools that you can use when you think it is appropriate.

Make sure that the patient knows what you are doing

The intention here is that the patient stays quiet while you are concentrating on the screen. You could just say 'Please be quiet while I do this', but there are more subtle ways of phrasing this, and many variations on the theme. If the words are accompanied by body movements, or a turning of the head, their impact will be greater. When we looked at videos of consultations, we often saw the GP building up to the transfer to the computer over several exchanges in the dialogue. The GP would, for example, use closed questions or leave shorter gaps before talking; this engineers a definite break in the dialogue.

Talk all the time you are using the computer, so that the patient cannot get a word in

The talk does not need to be very sophisticated! You can discuss the weather, gardening, sport or politics – anything that you can cover without having to think too deeply! An alternative is to give a running commentary on what you are doing on the computer. Some GPs just talk very slowly while they are using the computer. The effect of all these different tactics is the same: because you are talking and filling the space, it is difficult for the patient to start off on a different tack.

Use the computer without giving any verbal cues, but turn back to the patient every time they speak

This is very effective as a means of keeping rapport. It requires discipline to turn away from text that you are engaged in, but it can be done. In some ways it is just good manners: if the other person in the room is talking, you should listen properly.

Positioning the screen on the desk

If you are lucky, you can position your computer on the desk in what you think is the ideal place – relative to you and the patient. It may well be that you are working at someone else's desk, or that the room is designed in such a way that there is only one place to put the screen. You may be able to choose how things are, or you may have to make the best of the situation.

There are two main considerations here. One is 'How easy is it for the patient to see the screen?' The other is 'Do I have to move to use the computer?' If the screen is at the same end of the desk as the patient, and it is angled towards you, it is easy for you to glance from one to the other. One consequence of this is that it is harder for the patient to know where your attention is; the other consequence is that it is quite difficult for the patient to see the screen. If the screen is at the end of the desk away from the patient, it is much easier for them to read from it. This arrangement also means that you have to turn away from the patient in order to type or read from the screen. This is helpful as a way of communicating what you are doing, but it does make it harder for you to pick up cues from the patient since they are out of your sight.

Confidentiality and who can see the screen

Wherever the screen is placed in the room, it may well be visible to friends or relatives who come into the room with the patient. This can raise issues of confidentiality. There can also be problems if someone has typed contentious or unguarded comments in the patient's record, not expecting them to be seen by the patient.

There is also a big difference between writing a prescription under the eyes of the patient, and typing in a diagnosis, or being watched as you use an information source online. The prescription is an instruction to another professional: it describes a plan of action. Typing in a Read code, or being observed as you navigate round a decision-support program is much more of a disclosure: you are showing what you think and how your mind is working. Different practitioners at different times, with different patients and different problems, will feel more or less comfortable with sharing things in this way. Similarly, some patients will be keen to see what is on the screen and others will not really think that it is their business. Therefore, it is important for each practitioner to be aware of the consequences of different screen placements.

Using the computer in real consultations

So far in this chapter we have looked at knowledge flows in the consultation, some of the literature about computer use, described some skills that enable computer use and considered some of the consequences of the way equipment and furniture is arranged in the room. In this final section we will try to relate this abstract and theoretical approach to real consultations.

It is important to note that for many consultations computer use in the presence of the patient may be minimal. Reading the electronic record and summary before the patient comes into the room may provide all the information that the practitioner needs. During the consultation the practitioner can rely on experience and familiarity with common conditions, and knowledge of his or her patient. Then, as the consultation closes, a prescription or patient information leaflet can be printed out, providing a closure to the encounter.

Increasingly, as more records are kept online, there will be more need to scroll back through the electronic record to find previous entries, read letters from hospital consultants, or find laboratory results. As the continuing care of chronic conditions becomes more structured you may wish to fill in computerised templates while the patient is with you. Also, as more and more useful information is readily available and as patients (and practitioners) get used to the idea, referring to the computer for knowledge support will become commonplace. Even so, computer use of this sort will not be appropriate in every consultation. How do practitioners decide on when to use the computer? How do they negotiate this with their patients?

What does the patient think?

The work by Als,[4] and also a recent survey of patients in a training practice[9] shows that patients' attitude to computer use by their doctors varies considerably from one person to another. Whereas some people will welcome evidence that their doctor is up to date, others will be concerned that their doctor does not know all the answers.

What do I want to achieve?

Reference to the computer in the consultation has several different purposes. The task may be essential to the process of the consultation: for instance looking back at previous records for the sake of context, generating a prescription or recording data in a template. You may be using the computer as an optional alternative such as using the electronic version of the *British National Formulary* (*BNF*) to find out about the side effects of a drug rather than looking it up in the book version. You may even be using the computer as an additional resource, such as using a shared doctor–patient screen or a patient leaflet, to add weight to the advice you have given verbally.

Each of these tasks requires a different approach. Before using the computer in these ways you should consider:

- What am I trying to achieve by using the computer here?
- Does the patient understand what I am doing?
- What does this patient think about me using the computer in this way?
- Can I do this now without spoiling the rapport in the consultation?

More often that not, you will have a tacit understanding or intuition about the answers to these questions; sometimes you will have to ask directly. There are parallels here between shared understanding of the processes of the consultation and shared understanding of the patient's condition. Shared understanding of these processes has been shown to enhance rapport and improve outcomes, and shared understanding of the condition is known to improve compliance or concordance with treatment and to improve health. Encouragingly, it is also known that these skills can be taught and learnt.

Conclusion

In this chapter, we have introduced the idea of the triadic consultation – the GP, the patient and the computer. This raises important issues of how to maintain rapport and communication with the patient while using the computer to assist with the consultation. Practical tips to cope with these problems have been outlined. A CD-ROM, 'Using the Computer in the Consultation', which can be used as an educational and training tool, has been produced by the team at Sowerby Centre for Health Informatics – see the PRODIGY website (www.prodigy.nhs.uk).

References

1   Robinson PJ and Heywood P (2000) What do GPs need to know? The use of knowledge in general practice consultations. *British Journal of General Practice* **50**: 56–9.
2   Douglas C (1975) *The Houseman's Tale*. Cannongate Publishing, London.

3   Wilson R (1998) *Prodigy Phase Two – Use and Non-use of Prodigy Clinical Recommen-dations and Clinical Computers by Women GPs*. Sowerby Centre for Health Informatics, Newcastle upon Tyne.

4   Als AB (1997) The desk-top computer as a magic box: patterns of behaviour connected with the desk-top computer; GPs' and patients' perceptions. *Family Practice* **14**: 17–23.

5   Herzmark GA, Brownbridge G, Fitter M and Evans A (1984) Consultation use of a computer by general practitioners. *British Journal of General Practice* **34**: 649–54.

6   Warshawky SS, Pliskin JS, Urkin J *et al.* (1994) Physician use of a computerized medical record system during the patient encounter: a descriptive study. *Computer Methods Programs* **43**: 269–73.

7   Sullivan F and Mitchell E (1995) Has general practitioner computing made a difference to patient care? A systematic review of published reports. *BMJ* **311**: 848–52.

8   Greatbach D, Luff P, Heath C and Campion P (1993) Interpersonal communication and human–computer interaction: an examination of the use of computers in medical consultations. *Interacting with Computers* **5**: 193–216.

9   Garcia R (2002) Personal communication.

5

Teams working e-together

Louise Simpson

With the benefits of the technology that the NHS is gearing up to deliver to frontline staff, we will find ourselves part of a virtual team (or e-team) with members located in different parts of the country, in different organisations, in different professional groups, but all working with the same individual patient. We already belong to different horizontal working groups – the same speciality – and wider professional groups or communities of practice. All these types of groups and teams are in the spotlight here.

Thinking about what we want to do with all this technology is putting the cart well before the horse. The starting point is to be clear about the vision for healthcare. The extent to which we can influence the vision varies – it might be to change the whole shape of primary care and the way organisations structure themselves. This sort of first-order change usually spirals into the next round of reorganisation without the dust settling. More meaningfully, we must set a clear vision of the kind of healthcare service I want for my patients, my family, my own children and myself. This inspires the sort of second-order change that will affect the experience of patients when they encounter the practice and the practice team. What kind of team are we? What context do we work in? What can we do to achieve the vision we set for ourselves?

Setting the e-scene

Almost everyone working in the NHS has access to a desk-top or lap-top computer, and new hand-held devices are becoming popular. At home, a computer with access to the internet and e-mail is part of the furniture, and the supermarket delivery van is being kept busy by increasing numbers of online shoppers.

What does this mean for those of us at work in the NHS? Browsing information pages that hold the most up-to-date evidence-based guidance or the latest policy briefing is only part of the story. If I am online, so are many hundreds and thousands of others at the same time. And once I have switched my computer off, many thousands more will just be turning theirs on. These virtual networks mean people can be in touch with people from similar professional groups, interest groups and organisational groups without the need for large meetings and more time out from the day job. It also means that structured data entry into a patient-centred single electronic record (or a spine summary) becomes feasible and possible. The patient's narrative is available to those that need to know – the story will no longer be fragmented across a multitude of sites, departments and formats.

Starting at the beginning

Designing data entry fields for electronic records would be putting the cart well before the horse but this is often the starting point when different teams from different disciplines get together with the aim of working towards a single patient-centred record that different staff groups, from different teams in different organisations, can use together. The starting point should be to clarify the vision for healthcare and what care for a particular patient should look like.

The extent to which we can influence the vision varies – it might be to change the whole shape of primary care and the way organisations structure themselves, or it might be to do what we already do, but better.

There is still value in reviewing and refining what we do already, and the detail cannot be overlooked – patients being told to telephone after 4 pm on Monday for results that are not going to be available until Thursday is frustrating for patients and leads to anxiety and confusion for frontline desk staff, who may have six or seven interactions with a patient for every encounter between the patient and a member of the clinical team.

Decision-making for e-teams

Part of the reason teams come together is to make decisions. These decisions might be about the care of a patient, the organisation of a service or the development of a training strategy. A number of theories exist about how groups or teams reach decisions. Will groups make different decisions when they are 'virtual'? Will e-team decisions be as acceptable as current methods?

How teams make decisions

Stephen Littlejohn's book, *Theories of Human Communication*,[1] has a thorough chapter looking at how groups make decisions. He outlines Follett's ideas that group or team decision-making is a creative, three-fold process:[2]

- gathering information from experts
- testing that information in everyday experience
- developing integrative solutions that meet a variety of interests rather than competing among interests.

Computers are good at enabling access to information. The problem with them can lie in filtering the overload of information sources. For the purposes of making decisions about the care of an individual patient, access to the NHS Care Records Service, to a complete set of notes about the whole of a patient's health and illness record, will be a positive step. Its application in decision-making will depend on individual practitioners' trust in the data they are accessing, and in planning the context of the fullest possible picture of the patient.

Littlejohn writes:

> *Decision-making in a group is different from individual problem solving because of interpersonal relations. Whenever two or more people come together to handle a problem, interpersonal obstacles also arise. Such obstacles include the need to make your ideas clear to others, handle conflict, manage differences and so forth. Thus, in any group discussion, members will be dealing simultaneously with tasks and interpersonal obstacles.*[1]

Interpersonal play versus task focus

A balance between focussing on the task and dealing with the interpersonal issues is needed for a group or a team to function. Groups that focus too much on the task may not be confident and may be suffering from 'group-think' or power imbalances if there is no connection between their members – part of the reason for achieving connection is to achieve trust. Groups that spend too much time on interpersonal issues may also run the risk of group-think, and the risk of not being productive. Of course it may be that the purpose of the group is to network, and it may appear that interpersonal connections are the task itself, but most groups have a common goal and require synergy to achieve it.

How can the e-team pay attention to the interpersonal issues as well as the task in hand? First, it will be a challenge in the NHS Care Records Service to ensure that individual practitioners identify themselves as part of the e-team in the first place. Groups which meet in the same room have physical evidence of their 'team-ness' and still have a challenge in behaving like a team – this situation will be amplified in the virtual environment. Small digital photographs of e-team members, synchronous online discussions and occasional face-to-face meetings, where possible, can help to raise levels of trust and a sense of team-ness.

Group e-think

The 'group-think hypothesis' of Irving Janis is also thoroughly explored in Littlejohn's book,[1] and its notes on power and communication hold important messages for e-teams. Littlejohn notes that 'certain conditions can lead to high group satisfaction but ineffective output' and that 'group-think is a direct result of cohesiveness in groups'. With a sense of team that includes a high level of trust, accepting given information without critical appraisal can hinder critical, objective decision-making. Previous decisions are accepted, new hypotheses are accepted without criticism and the team's satisfaction with itself produces an unfounded level of confidence.

The following is Janis' toolkit to help recognise the characteristics of a team experiencing group-think and steps to prevent it.

- Encourage everyone to be a critical evaluator and express reservations whenever they come up.
- Do not have the leader state a preference up front.
- Set up several independent and separate policy-making groups.
- Divide the group into subgroups.
- Discuss what is happening with others outside the group.
- Invite insiders into the group to bring in fresh ideas.
- Assign an individual at each meeting to be devil's advocate.
- Spend considerable time surveying warning signals.
- Hold a second-chance meeting to reconsider decisions before making them final.

If a group's outcome depends on the quality of interactions within the group, and group-think is to be avoided when making decisions, how can the e-team ensure quality communications?

Communication skills for e-teams

The *Gower Handbook of Internal Communication*[3] offers a list of communication skills that are essential for teams working together:

- answering questions
- appearance
- appraisal
- asking questions
- assertiveness
- body language
- brainstorming
- briefing
- communicating through manuals and guides
- counselling
- delegating
- editing
- facilitating
- getting feedback
- giving feedback
- keeping it simple
- leading discussions
- letter, memo, fax and e-mail writing
- listening
- media management
- meetings
- negotiating
- networking
- neuro-linguistic programming (NLP)
- presentation
- reading
- report writing
- speaking
- speech and script writing
- summarising
- telephoning
- transactional analysis.

Working in an electronic world, in which handwriting is replaced by text on a screen, offers a new environment for all these skills. Patient-centred, intra-organisational electronic records will affect all of them, and the way teams work as a result.

None of the new technology will, or should, replace face-to-face meetings. Instead of the earlier situation, where face-to-face meetings could not always take place, now access to health events and encounter summaries will be available at the click of a button, regardless of location, time of day (midnight in the A&E department, for example) or staff group, subject to the appropriate confidentiality and security arrangements.

Let us take a look at a couple of items from the above list,[3] ... and ask some questions about how these important communication skills might evolve in the light of the NHS Care Records Service.

Delegating

Delegation implies an hierarchical issuing of instructions and in lots of instances this will be the case. But let us look at delegation in the wider sense: that different people in the primary care team offer different bits of the care package to the patient.

- Is the person to whom you are delegating a task available in the same building as you at the same time?
- What means are available to you now to pass on calls-for-action?
- What are the problems with this way of doing things?
- What duplication of effort or gaps arise?

Listening

So much communication is carried in the way we say things: the pauses between words, how we use our hands or nod our heads while speaking. Listening is an important clinical tool, but how can we listen when the communication media are electronic? We talk about 'reading between the lines' – can we still do this when the 'lines' are on a computer screen? Some of our ability to listen will depend on what the computer supplier has set up for us – do we have to search for information about a patient or about a new clinical guideline, or is it pushed to us as a prompt? Are the gaps in a clinical history prompted to us as well? Can the software allow us to look forwards and backwards along a medical storyline? Are the appropriate words – significant events and key clinical items – foregrounded rather than lost in a screen of 'same-font, same-size' text? The talent for 'listening' with our eyes will be ever more important in a computer-based clinical consultation or when reviewing electronic healthcare records.

Networking

Attending training events, clinical meetings or conferences is an important learning tool in order to glean the content of lectures and presentations. The coffee and lunch breaks, and breakout sessions are often the best bit, though: helping us to consolidate what we have heard in the 'taught' session and to network with our peers and colleagues. The e-world and the internet give us access to a worldwide network of peers. GP-UK (see www.gp-uk.org) is a well established electronic community of practice, and a plethora of others – both formal and informal – is available. Some e-communities will convene for a specific purpose and for a finite time period, for example to support a learning activity. Some will have a longer life, perhaps providing cohesion for colleagues at different geographic locations. Many specialist groups' websites give details of their e-community, or we can try a web search to gain access to one.

Report writing

Like it or not, report writing is an ever-increasing part of the business of primary care. Clinical reports and letters can be much less painful if the basics of data quality are right. Automated insurance reports and clinical summaries for referral letters rely on consistent coding and accurate data entry. However, the time saved in generating audits, reports, referral summaries and insurance reports is one of the key benefits of electronic health records for the busy practice team. It takes the same amount of time to enter the 'right' data during a consultation as to do 'off-road coding'. See www.primis.nhs.uk for more information about data quality education. Most primary care trusts now have information governance programmes which offer guidance on coding and information quality.

How teams might change

Taking on new ways of doing things

Guidance, best practice, protocols and other key messages can be cascaded much more quickly in the electronic environment. The lead time from completing a paper document to distributing a printed paper copy can be reduced dramatically by making an electronic copy available. More practically, too, real changes to practice can happen within hours of new guidance emerging – flags set on computer screens, field changes to templates and protocols, intranets highlighting the key points the next time you switch on your computer. New knowledge can be disseminated rapidly, although it is easily missed if e-mail distribution is the only e-communication tool used – e-mail volume seems to be a modern measure of stress for people in the workplace. There are opportunities, too, seeing the computer-based story of another colleague's approach to an encounter or condition can prompt reflection in a safe and non-threatening way.

Flatter structures

Paul Samuels writes that 'organisations ... no longer need a large number of middle managers controlling and often censoring information ... The new networks ensure information can reach anyone who needs it.'[4]

Of course this applies equally to patients who now have home access to an extraordinary quantity of health information of varying quality, but GPs are not seeing empty waiting rooms as a result. Similarly, middle layers of management in organisations are not being swept away, their roles and skills are changing. Patients need more support, not less, to filter and assimilate the paper mountain any search engine offers.

Issues for e-teams

The electronic domain offers new ways of working for teams that might be based in organisations, or networking opportunities to peers across disparate geographic areas. The core electronic healthcare record will be available across teams and organisations, following the story of the patient care process, and supporting single assessment and patient-centred information. Multi-agency and multidisciplinary teams will be able to access a common set of clinical data for decision-making.

The availability of a common clinical health record gives us a set of new challenges when relying on a data set for clinical and management decision-making.

Control over editing

We must be satisfied by the provider of the common electronic care record that the data are intact and reliable, and that editing, deleting and amending functions are accounted for and accountable. Electronic messages that make a change to a patient's core clinical record need to be attributed to an appropriate clinician – and access should depend on the most stringent of security and confidentiality procedures.

Bringing on the 'technophobes'

What constitutes an e-team? Is it the same as a 'regular' team? A team might be described as a group of people with a common goal. When the team caring for a patient over an extended period, whether in single or multiple episodes, is based in different departments, different buildings and different organisations, the traditional sense of a 'team' might not exist. Individuals might not recognise themselves as part of a wider team and thus might not 'sign up' to a common goal. The common goal might be to achieve a quality electronic medical record, so getting the technophobes involved will be a big challenge to the achievement of a multidisciplinary, patient-centred single care process.

Did I really mean to say that?

When writing a diary, it is often suggested that the author bears in mind that their diary might be read by other people. The same must be true of a medical record – few notes are for the author's eyes only, even with the most stringent of controls and security, and the electronic 'security' envelope. Bear this in mind when writing medical notes: your old scribbles in a 'Lloyd George' might well be transferred into the electronic record and made available to a consultant neurologist or obstetrician in an acute unit in another part of the country.

Wildly disparate coding systems and millions of codes

Handwritten notes are all 'free text', but many healthcare practitioners are now familiar with the concept of clinical coding and capturing quality information in electronic systems. However, with myriad different systems and millions of clinical codes from different coding systems, people within the same general practice sometimes find it challenging to adhere to a common scheme. The 'work streams' of the information governance programme go some way towards ensuring common understanding in a common core clinical electronic health record, but the technology must also support us in getting there.

Trust in the anonymous source of an entry into the patient record

Can I really trust a piece of information in a clinical record? Can I make a decision with a patient, based on data supplied from a person or team that I have no sense or knowledge of? How can I critically appraise information on which I am going to base my decisions?

These are all good and valid questions which are magnified by the way electronic health records will be developed and delivered under the NHS Care Records Service, but they are not exclusive to it. These themes of the role of information in doubt and uncertainty in decision-making are familiar to clinicians. The steps taken by clinical and administrative teams to ensure the provenance of information will be crucial to trust in e-records and e-teams.

Trust that someone will check their e-mail and e-records

Paper can be glanced at, Post-It notes can be placed strategically on chairs or keyboards, but there is no guarantee that individuals will check their e-mail for urgent messages. However, the benefit of a single record, a single source for data representing a patient, means that an opportunity exists to concentrate on this problem.

A final thought

A common identity, a clear objective and an appropriate task balanced with taking care of interpersonal issues are required from groups and teams making decisions. When the group is a virtual one, its members risk seeing themselves as part of a *process*, but not necessarily as part of a *team*. The advent of new clinical information systems, which cross time and place, offers a new set of issues for consideration. Encouraging a sense of 'teamness' is an important factor in our use of the electronic care records service.

References

1   Littlejohn S (2002) *Theories of Human Communication.* Wadsworth, London.
2   Follett MP (1924) *Creative Experience.* Longman Green & Co., New York.
3   Newbold A and Scholes E (1997) *Gower Handbook of Internal Communication.* Gower, London.
4   Samuels P (1998) The impact of computer-based communication's network. In: E Scholes (ed.) *The Gower Handbook of Internal Communication.* Gower Publishing, Aldershot.

6

Information governance

Rob Wilson

What is information governance?

There is long-standing confusion caused by the legislation, records management guidance, security and confidentiality policies that apply to the NHS. The concept of information governance intends to offer an appropriate means by which to support compliance with existing legislation and good information confidentiality and security practice in the NHS. It has been defined as:

> *a framework which aims to support organisations and individuals in the NHS to ensure that personal information is dealt with legally, securely, efficiently and effectively, in order to deliver the best possible care.*[1]

The concept of information governance incorporates the HORUS standards (Holding, Obtaining, Recording, Using and Sharing), expanded below:

- *holding* information securely and confidentially
- *obtaining* information fairly and efficiently
- *recording* information accurately and reliably
- *using* information effectively and ethically
- *sharing* information appropriately and lawfully.

The HORUS standards were subsequently turned into a framework by adding an axis which allowed categories to be applied to the variety of available materials (management, systems, processes and people), shown in Table 6.1.

Table 6.1 The HORUS framework

	Holding	Obtaining	Recording	Using	Sharing
Management	Structures Policies and procedures	Structures Policies and procedures	Structures Policies and procedures	Structures Policies and procedures	Structures Policies and procedures
Systems	Access controls Cryptography Monitoring/audit Remote working	N/A	Application security Validation Audit of data input	N/A	N/A
Processes	Systems support Physical/ environment Operational procedures Personnel security Compliance/review	Compliance/review Protocols (receipt) Informing patients/ clients Caldicott processes	Data quality assurance System design Compliance/ review Records management	IM&T controls Caldicott processes Availability of records Compliance/review	Subject access Compliance/ review Lawful disclosure Protocols (disclosure)
People	ETD Guidance	Guidance ETD	Guidance ETD	Guidance ETD	Guidance ETD

ETD = Education, training and development

Why is information governance important?

There are many apocryphal tales of how easy it is to obtain sensitive medical information, either by deception or through incompetence. For instance, I used to travel on a minibus shuttle service which ran between two hospitals, and which was also used for the transit of medical records, X-rays and test results. So it appears to be a relatively simple process to obtain confidential information from the NHS, and this threat is real. Second, and most important, is that this situation could happen to anyone: of the thousands of people who work for the NHS, those same people are also its patients. It is in everybody's interest to ensure that high-quality information practice is the norm.

What are the aims of information governance?

The national programme for information governance has four aims.

- To support the provision of high-quality care by promoting the effective and appropriate use of information.
- To encourage responsible staff to work closely together, preventing duplication of effort and enabling more efficient use of resources.
- To develop support arrangements and provide staff with appropriate tools and support to enable them to discharge their responsibilities to consistently high standards.
- To enable organisations to understand their own performance and manage improvement in a systematic and effective way.[1]

These aims were devised to highlight and support the implementation of information governance practice in organisations across the NHS within the general modernisation agenda initiated by *The NHS Plan*,[2] the work of the NHS Modernisation Agency and the implementation of the NHS National Programme for Information Technology.

What are the requirements for primary care?

Overall, the aims are being supported by the provision of a number of resources (including the information governance toolkit)[3] and varying degrees of encouragement. At the time of writing the situation is that acute trusts will be *mandated* to use the toolkit, primary care trusts will be *required* to use it and GPs will be *encouraged* to use it. It is likely, however, that primary care trusts may be mandated to use the toolkit in the future.

However, its requirements are not arduous and many of them fall into the category of good practice.

A number of strategic health authorities and primary care trusts have begun to focus on the information governance agenda and are co-ordinating their efforts. A good point of contact for local developments should be the organisation's appointed Caldicott Guardian. The professional bodies of general practitioners (see below) have also responded to the agenda and have produced documentation which describes in some detail the requirements for general practices. A discussion and summaries of some of the requirements for the various stakeholders may be found below, divided into organisations and roles.

How can we *do* information governance in general practice?

There is a set of roles and responsibilities for strategic health authorities and primary care trusts in the development and implementation of information governance. The initial steps in the process should include the appointment of senior manager(s), with board-level responsibility for information governance, and establishing a steering group and nominated lead to take forward operational or practical issues. General practices also need to respond to the day-to-day concerns of caring for their patients' information. Guidance for general practice is set out in the publication of the joint computing group of the General Practitioner Committee and the Royal College of General Practitioners, *Good Practice Guidelines for General Practice Electronic Patient Records* (version 3).[4] In summary, the guidance on information governance recommends that:

- practices must have a mechanism for giving patients access to their records on request
- practices should consider giving patients access to their records routinely at some point in the process of care to validate them
- practices should only share patient information with the consent of the patient
- informed consent may be deemed both ethically and legally to be implied but [a number of] principles should apply for this to be the case, including, for example, the applications of consent to a 'defined local health network' and the exceptions to consent, such as a 'statutory notification of a disease'.

Further recommendations set out a series of policies and processes that should be produced and undertaken by general practices, including arrangements to cover risk management, accessibility, capacity and storage, physical security, access control, security policy, disposal and IT recovery arrangements.

What resources are available?

As well as the local guidance and resources outlined above, the information governance toolkit[3] is the main resource available to support the implementation of information governance. The aim of the toolkit is to fulfil the following objectives.

- Supporting NHS employees to manage personal information for the benefit of the patient or client.
- To provide a framework to bring together all the requirements, standards and best practice which applies to handling personal information.
- To set standards and give organisations the tools to achieve them.

Some documents are available on the NHS Information Authority website (www.nhsia.nhs.uk). Contact the help desk by telephone (0121 333 0420) or by e-mail (helpdesk3@nhsia.nhs.uk).

Final thoughts

There are clear advantages to adopting an NHS-wide approach to governing information. It allows the NHS, and its many parts, to demonstrate that it is learning from the past in its approach to the processing and use of information about patients.

Information governance is the beginning of a continuous process to address the long-standing challenge of providing a framework to support the principles of security and confidentiality in the NHS. The information governance toolkit and the corresponding HORUS model offer a starting point from which to understand, navigate and operate the policy documents and legislation that have been put in place in over the years. They also offer a way to audit activity and progress at an organisational level. However, this is only the starting point, and we have a clear requirement to sustain this work over an extended period. It is fair to say that information is not always treated with due care and attention within the NHS, and that the culture change needed to bring about an appropriate change in caring information practice by NHS employees should not be underestimated.

References

1   NHS Information Authority (2004). http://www/nhsia.nhs.uk (accessed December 2004).
2   Department of Health (2000) *The NHS Plan*. Department of Health, London.
3   *The Information Governance Toolkit*. www.nhsa.nhs.uk/infogov.igt
4   General Practitioner Committee and the Royal College of General Practitioners (2003) *Good Practice Guidelines for General Practice Electronic Patient Records* (Version 3). GPC–RCGP, London.

7

Health inequalities and language diversity

Mark Gibson and Pam Turpin

This chapter looks at how the primary care team can use technology to bolster care in multilingual settings.

Language diversity, health inequalities and patient information provision

Although there are no official figures relating to the languages spoken in the UK, it is estimated that approximately 5% of the population speaks a native language other than English. In London alone, approximately 310 languages are represented by its diverse population, and many groups within our black and ethnic minority communities have little or limited knowledge of English. Therefore, GPs in many areas are bound to encounter patients who speak a language other than English.

Although the distribution of the languages spoken throughout the UK resembles a hugely complex sociolinguistic mosaic, the dominant community languages in the UK can be classified, in crude terms, into five discrete categories.

- *Native*: languages that are native to the British Isles and precede the arrival and development of English, such as Welsh and Scottish Gaelic.

- *Nativised*: languages introduced by communities established in the UK, in some cases for well over a century, such as Urdu, Punjabi, Gujarati, Mirpuri, Bengali, Cantonese, Turkish and Greek.
- *Recent*: languages introduced by relatively recent waves of settlers and asylum seekers, such as Arabic, Kurdish, Farsi, Somali and Albanian.
- *Auxiliary*: languages used worldwide, and spoken in the UK, such as Hindi, French, Spanish, Portuguese and Russian.
- *Tourism*: languages spoken by people who visit the UK annually in large numbers, such as Japanese and Italian, as well as the auxiliary languages mentioned above.

To place language diversity into a healthcare context, it is well documented that people belonging to the black and ethnic minority communities face a shorter life expectancy and poorer physical and mental health than the general UK population. It is an epidemiological fact that people of Pakistani, Indian and Bangladeshi origins, for instance, have a greater chance of developing a chronic illness such as diabetes, heart disease or low blood pressure, whereas smoking cessation on a national scale is lowest among older males within these communities. It is also claimed that half of the Pakistani and Bangladeshi households in the UK have no income from employment.[1] Further, sustained institutional discrimination is directly related to the prevalence of clinical depression and associated mental health conditions among people from the black and ethnic minority communities.[1]

The black and ethnic mintority patient populations struggle with a health service that is poorly equipped to deal with individual cultural and religious needs. More pertinently, language is cited as a chief barrier to many patients who attempt to access primary care services. However, it is ironic that although, as an annual average, people of South Asian origin visit their GPs more than the mainstream population, these perceived healthcare inequalities continue to persist.[2] It is also claimed that, in Leicester, patients of South Asian origin suffering ischaemic heart disease regularly wait longer for referrals in cardiology clinics when compared to white patients.[3] In addition, although a relatively high proportion of Leicester's population is of South Asian origin, it has been found that South Asian patients report more problems in gaining access to their GPs than non-Asian patients.[4]

It is reported that people who have limited knowledge of English are often given less healthcare or condition-specific information, whether written or verbal, from their GPs.[1] Furthermore, since there are no real feedback processes in place for speakers of languages other than English, these patients believe they are kept 'out of the loop' of UK healthcare planning.[1] This sentiment may be especially apparent among recent settlers in the UK, for example refugees and asylum seekers.[5] Therefore, the result of such exclusion on the basis of ethnicity and linguistic competence is poorly treated conditions, increased morbidity and mortality, and, ultimately, wasted time and money for the Department of Health.

Paradoxically, within the current climate of 'empowerment' among the general patient population, there is a chronic marginalisation of black and ethnic minority patients on a nationwide scale. These inequalities have been highlighted by healthcare professionals for many years and were briefly discussed in the 1998 Green Paper, *Our Healthier Nation*,[6] published by the Department of Health, as well as almost myriad other documents since, such as *Electronic Health Horizons*.[7]

Now, to help cater for black and ethnic minority communities' healthcare requirements, all primary care trusts and primary caregivers have at least one health inequalities or diversity officer. In addition, GPs have access to community language interpreters and liaison officers, and often have stocks of leaflets in various languages, covering a wide range of conditions and lifestyle issues.

However, it is a notorious fact that interpreters may not always be readily available and, rather than offering healthcare for patients, a large volume of preprinted leaflets provide 'shelf-care' in practice waiting rooms, since translations may not be socioculturally sensitive, may be difficult to understand and their clinical content may not always be evidence-based. This kind of written information provided in community languages may be rejected by patients.

There are practicalities to providing public services such as multilingual patient information, and these merit consideration. With more than 300 languages represented in the UK, a key question is which languages would be eligible for translation. The demand for translation appears to be recognised in terms of speaker numbers and community need. Clearly, it is relatively easy to address the former by means of identifying those community languages that are more numerically dominant. Ideally, these would include languages such as Urdu, Punjabi, Hindi, Cantonese, and so forth.

However, individual and community need may be more difficult to identify. For instance, although represented in fewer numbers in the UK, patient information in Somali, Kurdish, Pushtu and Romany is evidently required in an attempt to bolster primary care for patients currently seeking asylum in the UK.[5,8]

In addition, other issues come into play when planning patient information in general practice. For example, many speakers of other languages in the UK have ancestral links with regions which are culturally and linguistically complex. This is reflected in speakers' linguistic repertoires in the UK. Accordingly, the question of which language should be addressed becomes relevant. To target the Bangladeshi community, should health information be rendered in Sylheti or Bengali? Opting for the former would mean that the information should be in audio or audiovisual format, since

Sylheti does not have a written form. A sizeable section of the Pakistani population in a city such as Bradford speaks both Punjabi, Mirpuri and Urdu, yet may read only English. Many citizens of Indian origin speak Gujarati or Punjabi rather than Hindi, yet audio recordings of Hindi may be a more practical language for health information translation owing to its status as a South Asian and British Asian lingua franca.

Wilson recommends that English language patient information leaflets should be aimed at a readability level of 12 years old to achieve maximum and effective dissemination of the message.[9] Furthermore, as with information provision in English, patient information leaflets provided in community languages ought to be relevant, easy to understand and accessible. However, Hawthorne states that many translated leaflets are direct translations from English and relate to an 'English' way of life, sometimes full of grammatical and spelling errors. In addition, without sustained research on a national basis, it is difficult to estimate the literacy competences of speakers of community languages.[3] For example, it should not even be assumed that speakers are literate in their respective languages. Hawthorne reports that in Blackburn 11% of Gujarati speakers and 26% of Punjabi speakers could not read or write their respective languages.[3] So, another key question should be whether this information ought to be provided in audio, audiovisual or written versions.

How can technology help?

Internet and information provision is a key tool in this field. Of course, GPs and health service researchers across the UK have long been aware of health inequalities, and they have not only sought a potential solution in technology but have also decided to find one for themselves, often using their own resources and finances. Consequently, there are a number of free multilingual resources for GPs, mostly created by GPs, which can be accessed online, selected for the patient or carer in the relevant language and printed out accordingly.

An obvious example of this is the mypil.com website (www.mypil.com). This resource was created by a small number of GPs based in the north of England and it is dedicated to improving patient care by providing healthcare professionals with accessible, quality information about health-related and lifestyle issues. Although only four languages are currently represented on the website – English, Hindi, Urdu and Bengali – its potential for expansion is massive as more conditions and languages can be added to it.

Similarly, another resource (www.patient.co.uk) offers more than 500 evidence-based, validated leaflets on healthcare and lifestyle issues, which GPs can print out for their patients. Currently, only one leaflet is available in a language other than English (asthma, in Bengali) but more are planned for the future. At the same time, it should not be forgotten that English, too, is a dominant community language in the UK, and English speakers also require simple, quality healthcare information.

Another useful resource is the lottery-funded London Advice Services Alliance's (LASA) multikulti project (www.multikulti.org.uk), providing culturally appropriate and accurately translated advice and information in 11 of the dominant UK community languages, which deals with practical social subjects for newcomers to the UK.

Also, although not an online resource, the Minority Ethnic Health Awareness (MEHA) Project UK, funded by the Department of Health, provides information in community languages of South Asian and Middle Eastern origin in book, CD-ROM and video cassette formats. The Health for Asylum Seekers and Refugees Portal (HARP) (www.harpweb.co.uk) is a massive resource, a feature of which is a multilingual appointment card, which issues appointment booking information in 31 languages. These two projects appear to be the only nationwide initiatives receiving public funding.

Another option is the NHS Direct website (www.nhsdirect.nhs.uk/audio.asp), which offers sound bytes and audio clips of condition-specific and lifestyle advice in languages such as English, Punjabi, Gujerati and Bengali. Initiatives such as multilingual audio clip files found on the NHS Direct website are a sensible way of addressing the literacy issues mentioned above. However, such a facility assumes that patients not only have access to the internet, but also have the multimedia software packages needed to put this information to its fullest use. This is not often the case. It is estimated that although more than two-thirds of the UK population are regular users of the internet, the 'digital divide' between the IT 'haves' and the IT 'have-nots' is perceptible. In a UK context, there is little evidence to suggest a correlation between race, ethnicity, linguistic competence and access to technology.[7]

HARP links a lot of its information to the impressive New South Wales Multicultural Health Communication Service in Australia (www.mhcs.health.nsw.gov.au), which is funded by the New South Wales Health Authority, and which provides information and advice for dozens of conditions in 46 languages, many of which are languages that are relatively new in the UK, yet are still spoken in large numbers in the UK by recent asylum seekers (such as Kurdish and Somali).

Conclusion

Websites such as those discussed in this chapter provide a means of reducing potential costs: it is becoming increasingly apparent the internet is an ideal vehicle for the deployment of public multilingual information. For example, at the click of a mouse, it is possible to render the majority of the contents of the National Assembly for Wales and the Scottish Parliament websites in Welsh and Scottish Gaelic, respectively. Similarly, these web-enabled resources have the potential of providing free information in as many languages as possible and on as many healthcare and lifestyle topics as demand dictates.

In Chapter 12 of this book the reader will find a case study of people with sight loss, of South Asian origin, in Bradford.

References

1   Henley A and Schott J (1999) Culture, Religion and Patient Care in a Multi-Ethnic Society: A handbook for professionals. Age Concern, London.

2   Bennett L, Qutub B and Bellis M (1998) Improving the Health of Black and Ethnic Minority Communities: A North West of England perspective. University of Liverpool, Liverpool.

3   Hawthorne K (1994) Accessibility and use of health care services in the British Asian Community. *Family Practice* **11**(4): 452–8.

4   Rashid A and Jagger C (1992) Attitudes to and perceived use of healthcare services among Asian and non-Asian patients in Leicester. *Br G Gen Pract* **42**.

5   Hargreaves S, Holmes A and Friedland JS (2000) Refugees, asylum seekers and general practice: room for improvement? *Br J Med Pract* **July**(2): 531–2.

6   Department of Health (1998) *Our Healthier Nation: A contract for health.* Green Paper. Department of Health, London.

7   Purves I, Wilson R and Gibson M (2000) *Electronic Health Horizons.* NHS Executive IPU. SCHIN, Newcastle.

8   Lehti A and Mattson B (2001) Health attitude to care and pattern of attendance among gypsy women – a general practice perspective. *Family Practice* **18**(4): 445–8.

9   Wilson R, Kenny T, Clark J *et al.* (1998) PILs Project Report. Ensuring the Readability, Understandability and Efficacy of the Phase 2 Prodigy Non-Drug Advice Leaflets/PILs. NHS Executive, Newcastle.

Part 3:
Practical matters

8

Diagnosing the problem and finding a solution

Mark Fletcher

How many times have you heard the phrase, 'communication is a good thing'? It may be so, but then again, it may not. How do we judge? The underlying assumption of this chapter is simple: communication is a good thing if it helps you to achieve what you are trying to achieve.

If we think, uncritically, that all communication is good, this chapter may disappoint you. There is an unerring pragmatism embedded in this part of the book: communication is a practical tool that may be used to help us to achieve the outcomes that we want. The outcomes themselves only become relevant when we start to look at the problems that we face. So, before we start to communicate anything, to anyone, through any channels, in any way, we need to understand the nature of the problem that we are dealing with.

What is the problem?

Perhaps this is easier to elicit in medicine than it is in everyday life. A patient comes into the surgery and says, 'I have a pain here.' The patient points to a part of the body and we make a judgement, based upon what it could be in the context of the patient's medical history, what conditions are prevalent at the time, what we know of their ability to describe conditions adequately and so forth.

Communication as a problem-solving tool is a different matter altogether. Typically, senior staff will say, 'We need an internal communications strategy.' Why? Just as a doctor might say 'Why?' to a patient who says, 'I need pain killers', we must ascertain how creating a long, relatively boring document will help anyone in an organisation. Frequently, the 'Why?' is very revealing. It may turn out that the reason that senior staff believe they need such a thing is because others expect it of them. The trust may be inspected and if there is no internal communications strategy in place – a document that senior staff can refer to – the organisation will be found wanting.

The problem is one of symbolism, in the first instance, rather than action.

Internal communications are important. It is vital that those who work in your organisation understand where the organisation is going and what their role in that process is. However, that is not necessarily the same thing as having a communications strategy and discussions with senior staff will frequently reveal that there are internal cultural issues that need to be dealt with. The idea that all these matters be resolved by creating a document and having the Board note, or agree, it is naïve. Communications are only part of the solution to a problem. Even now the problem – cultural issues – is no clearer. The real risk in assuming that we can wave a 'communications wand' is that we ignore the real situation. If communications are to be part of a solution to anything at all, we need to begin by defining the problem.

If one of the reasons that we are leafing through this book is that we believe that somehow it will provide us with answers to some of the challenges we face, then put the book down and write out a short list of the problems that we think it will help with. Once we have done that, we should share them with our colleagues and ask them to confirm our diagnosis.

What is the likely solution?

Increasingly, in medicine, solutions to problems can be tested. Evidence-based medicine has existed for many years. However, the same discipline is not always present in communications thinking. The paucity of diagnoses, the lack of evidence and poor evaluation, coupled with the notion that only communications experts can help solve such problems all combine to reinforce the idea that this kind of activity is akin to some kind of witchcraft.

To put things simply: before we can solve a problem – whatever it is – we have to know what will work and what will not. In this book we will be exposed to a range of possible solutions. And because of the nature of this publication we might be tempted to conclude that e-communication is the answer to whatever questions we might have. It is not. Indeed, in many situations sending out messages electronically may make things worse.

Take a typical problem: 'Our staff don't know what we're about.' The solution might, at first, appear to be a straightforward communications action: 'We'll tell them – then they'll know.'

Fine so far – until we try to write down exactly what we do. Readers will not be surprised to learn that much of what we say we do will be expressed in a language that few outside their managerial circles actually speak. Even if we can express our function in everyday language, it may be so strategic and wide-ranging that it is meaningless to our staff. Add to that, the fact that we may tell them what we do, but they may not hear us. We may put our case to the staff repeatedly, but your actions may simply bore them. The outcome may be that our staff, despite our best efforts, may be no better informed than if we had done nothing at all.

Some of these problems will be covered in greater depth in Chapter 9, but, to return to the problem, 'Our staff don't know what we're about', is that actually the case? If we work in primary care, do they not know that, basically, 'We make people who are ill better and help those who are well to stay well'? And, if that is the case, what is the problem?

If it is not the case, might it be that the way we have described the problem actually masks the real issue. For example, it may be that we are about to be inspected for the 'Investors in People' award and our vision statement explains in long, complex terms (making appropriate references to government initiatives and targets) exactly what our aspirations are. Success in the assessment may depend upon our staff being able to repeat these phrases in a way that suggests they both understand them and are acting upon them.

The problem here is a different one. Here, the solution may lie in promoting our key aims rigorously and ruthlessly, through various media, over a period of months. But other actions will be essential: we have to ensure that every member of our staff is able to make the link between what they do and the overall aims of the organisation. And here our overall aims may be questionable. For example, if we assert that we want to 'improve the health of the community' without saying which parts, how and when, our staff might either believe this aim to be no more than a 'pipedream'. Or worse, unachievable.

Crucially, communications is one of a number of problem-solving tools that will only work if we are clear about the nature of the problem we are facing and about the other actions we are planning to take to bring about a clear outcome.

Making it happen

It may be that we are very clear about the solutions to many of the communications problems we face. However, there may be other reasons why these solutions are not implemented.

Some questions to consider:

- Do we have the skills to implement the solution?
- Do we have the time?
- Do we have the resources?
- Do we have the will?
- Do we believe that the problems as described are the real problems?

Or, taking this thinking a stage further, we may conclude that the problems with communications are actually hiding more fundamental concerns that our practice faces. We may, for example, believe that we are seen in a negative light by colleagues in other practices or in the primary care trust or in the strategic health authority, or even further afield. We may believe that this is simply because we are poor at communicating our purpose.

However, it may be that these audiences are entirely aware of what we are 'about', but the reason that we are detecting antipathy from them may be because they simply do not like what we do.

One way to establish how our practice is seen is to carry out – or to commission – a 'reputation audit'. This is a simple survey which is designed to enable key stakeholders to describe us to a third party in an honest way. In reality, this is a way to tackle problems that we face, rather than believing that producing an e-bulletin will solve all our problems.

A typical reputation audit

Ideally, we should identify the key stakeholders: those who matter to our organisation. These are the people whose support we depend upon. We would then commission research to establish answers to the following questions.

- Are you aware of xxxx (your organisation)?
- What makes you aware of it?
- What do you think it does?
- On a scale of 1–10 (where 10 is excellent) how well do you think it delivers?
- On what basis do you make judgements about this organisation?
- Do you know the names of any of the key staff?
- What three words best sum up this organisation to you?

The results of the reputation audit will tell us whether the problems we face lie in the area of communications or are altogether more complex. The same technique can be applied to other audiences, such as staff, local people, patients and so forth.

9

Writing an e-communications strategy

Mark Fletcher

In earlier parts of this book we have read of communication as an activity in which one party is able to confirm that a second party has confirmed that a message has been received because the first party has received feedback. In this context, communication is an act that is principally about the transfer of information from one party to another. This chapter is designed to take that notion a stage further: communication is a purposeful activity intended to achieve specific outcomes.

We do not always communicate with people to inform them. Frequently, and in particular in a clinical setting, we communicate in order to bring about other outcomes. These may have less to do with what people *know* and more to do with how they might *feel*. We may want someone to feel reassured, less anxious or better. Thus, the way that we communicate, our choice of words and phrases, the tone of voice that we choose, the rate at which we are able to deliver the message, will have an effect on those feelings. So, the starting point for any e-communication strategy must be the desired outcome: what is our communication designed to achieve?

What is the starting point?

The answer to this question may seem blatantly obvious but it is often ignored: we need to know what our starting point is before we can plan our communication.

In the clinical setting, diagnosis is a crucial first step. Somehow, this notion escapes us when we communicate. We make relatively simple mistakes. We assume that people will know what we are talking about before we start communicating. Frequently, they do not.

We assume that others will be interested in our material because we are. Often not. We assume that we are communicating in a language that others will readily understand because we understand it. Wrong. We use jargon. Nothing is more offputting than words and concepts that leave us bewildered.

We may even assume that the things which we believe establish our credibility in the eyes of others have meaning for them: 'I write to you as the Director of Clinical Governance from Blankshire PCT.' So what? Most of that sentence will mean nothing to many people.

And, of course, if we base our communication on a false premise, we should not be surprised if much of what we say is ignored, misunderstood or misinterpreted. In other words, we precipitate a communications breakdown through our actions.

What can we do about it?

The answer is very simple. We need to establish a number of things before we undertake any communication with an audience we do not know.

- Who is our audience?
- What does our audience understand about us?
- How does our audience see the world?
- What is the easiest way to engage our audience?
- What is the preferred way of communicating to our audience?

Once we have a starting point – and that may be a bit surprising – we can begin the process of engagement. Why surprising? It may emerge that we know very little about our potential audience. It may also be the case that our audience has little, or no, idea about us. Our audience may see the world entirely differently – their concerns may be a million miles away from our understanding of the world. We may even not be able to engage our audience. And the preferred way of communicating may not be one we are comfortable with.

It may be that we are communicating with an audience which does not read, is not interested in posters and other forms of simple communications and will only be interested in what we have to say if we sit down and meet them face to face, which is a very time-consuming business.

Outcomes

It is important to be clear from the outset about what we are trying to achieve through our e-communications strategy. It is vital that we are honest at this point. It may be tempting to write down the things we feel ought to be part of our e-communications strategy. Here, we might include all sorts of phrases designed, in truth, to help *us* rather than our staff or our patients.

The clearer we are about the outcome we are trying to achieve the easier it will be to assess whether or not we are likely to succeed. For example, we may determine that 'electronic communications should be the principal source of news and information for staff within the practice'. In other words, if it really matters we will read it first in an e-mail from the practice manager.

Straightaway, we appreciate the complexities which arise from that statement. First, some people may not have access to e-mail. Or, if they do have access to e-mail, it may be via a shared computer at work. Second, our staff may rely upon conversations over coffee as a way of finding out what counts. This may work more effectively since the staff may find that they trust specific people to know what is really going on.

Third, the statement assumes that one person may know what is going on, or will be able to find out. It also assumes that there is one version of reality – in which everyone shares the same understanding of the events and activities that affect our practice. Fourth, the statement assumes that people will want to receive this information electronically when, really, some information – the stuff that really matters – needs to be delivered face to face. It is far more challenging to give out sensitive information electronically than it ever is when we are standing before someone to whom you have to give bad news.

Lastly, the statement assumes that we want to write down what we might want to say. The Freedom of Information Act, which came into force in January 2005, makes anything we write down electronically capable of being captured. Added to that, we are likely to rephrase difficult messages if we are forced to put them in writing – and we quickly become conscious that, taken out of context, our messages could do more harm than good, in particular to ourselves.

All of the above leads back to one key question: if we intend to communicate electronically, what do we hope to achieve that we would not be able to achieve otherwise?

It is worth raising this challenge at this point since we might otherwise be in danger of assuming that electronic communication is always a good thing. However, if we look at the some of the unintended outcomes arising from electronic communications, we might decide that it is not.

An example

The Dimbelby Medical Centre is a forward-thinking practice which has appointed one of its senior partners to lead on e-communication. Dr Smith's colleagues feel that he is equipped for the job since he always has the latest electronic equipment. An early-adopter, he was first to have a mobile phone, first to own a personal data assistant (he migrated quickly from a Psion to a Palm Pilot) and had Blackberry long before his colleagues at the Strategic Health Authority.

The practice has not discussed its e-policy and has delegated any decisions to Dr Smith since he always seems to know what needs to be done. Dr Smith has recently observed that senior health managers and policy makers are almost completely dependent upon Blackberries. He finds this to be the case since the only way he can communicate with them is via these devices – they do not return telephone calls and nobody uses letters any more. As a result, at a practice meeting Dr Smith recommends that all the partners and clinical staff now adopt Blackberries as the means through which they will communicate.

In Blackberry Month One everyone is happy with the new devices since they act as telephones, diaries and keep all e-mail in one place. By Month Two it is clear that many partners are addicted to their electronic support devices. Cases that were formerly discussed at meetings are now being handled between colleagues electronically. This, it is argued, allows for a quicker exchange of views as well as (it is thought by some) being able to keep a clear record of all transactions, in particular concerning difficult cases.

Then some unintended outcomes start to occur. First, the communication does not stop when the practice closes. Colleagues report e-mails arriving on Sunday mornings, which they feel compelled to respond to. Some are comfortable with this, others are not. The aggrieved parties ask for this situation to be raised under e-communications policy and want clear protocols stating when e-mail should and should not be sent.

Next, some colleagues report feeling excluded from clinical discussions. Previously, cases had been discussed openly at practice meetings. Now, many discussions have taken place online and simply do not appear on meeting agendas. Or, when they are discussed, some people seem to be better-informed than others (those who were not privy to earlier electronic discussions) and this leads to a sense that there are two tiers within the practice.

Third, some colleagues have adopted the practice of blind carbon copying (bcc) so that they can see the nature of discussions about difficult cases without the recipients of the e-mails knowing about this. This makes the colleagues feel both anxious and collusive. Anxious because they now need to remember what they have heard from whom privately and they do not want to have to worry about such subtleties. Collusive because they feel that their honesty and openness has been compromised by the assumptions that others are making about the way they are likely to want to behave.

Fourth, within weeks all users report that they have become addicted to e-mail and find that, despite the fact that their devices are always on, they feel the need to check repeatedly for new correspondence. Some are positive about this. Again, others are less so.

Finally, the practice e-champion, Dr Smith, is beginning to feel uneasy in his role and is considering giving it up since he feels that he is being blamed (wrongly) for the consequences of this new policy.

In short, the unintended outcomes could potentially interfere with the day-to-day running of the practice and its clinical efficiency.

Key points

- Be clear about the outcomes we intend to achieve with our e-communications strategy – before we implement it.

- Ensure, by checking with others who have undertaken this work, that our outcomes are *achievable*.

- Ensure that the outcomes are *desirable*.

- Look at other factors which might directly affect our ability to create this outcome.

- Discuss the implications with colleagues to ensure that they are knowingly involved in the process.

- Look at both the risks and benefits arising from the desired outcomes.

Audiences

If we look back to the Shannon model in Chapter 3, we will see that communication takes place between two parties. We all know that the real world is more complex. To begin with, both parties need to *want* to communicate with each other. But, even when they do, both parties need to share the same frame of reference. For communication to be as intended, the text that one party utters needs to be heard and received in the same terms as those in which it was spoken. It needs to mean the same as it was intended to.

Life is rarely so simple. Here, we focus on the notion of the audience: distinct groups of people who see the world in different ways from other distinct groups of people.

When putting together our e-communications strategy, we should be clear about the audiences with whom we are communicating. This will be more pertinent for primary care since, increasingly, we will be communicating with diverse groups of people, many of whom will not only see the world quite differently from traditional primary care staff but who will also describe it differently, too.

Here are some questions we need to think about.

Which audience are we communicating with?

Communication often fails because we do not differentiate between one audience and another one, and we make the mistake of thinking that what works for one audience will automatically work for another. Or we assume that the people we are communicating with see the world as we do (when they do not or cannot) and convey our message in language and concepts that they do not understand or are unfamiliar with.

What do we, as a practice, know about the audience?

In all likelihood, collectively, we know a great deal about many of the audiences that we need to communicate with. But do we share that knowledge? In practical terms, how will our colleagues be able to access information about a recipient in ways that enable them to take account of the collective knowledge the practice may have?

How does this audience see the world?

We should be clear about how this audience sees the world. It may be that the audience shares a common professional background. This could condition the way that the audience interprets the world. Just as doctors may view the world through the frame of differential diagnoses and a problem-solving approach, so other professions may understand reality through their own interpretive frameworks. Knowing who the audience is will make a difference.

Which words and concepts does the audience use to describe the world?

One way of ensuring that we connect with an audience (or, in the case of e-mail, a particular individual) is to use language with which the recipient feels comfortable. This is not intended to sound patronising. Unless we are clear about how the person we are talking to constructs the world in their mind, we will find it harder to engage that person.

At its most basic, this question is about recognising that many of the terms which clinical staff take for granted will be meaningless to members of the public. For many people, the use of medical terms might simply reassure them that doctors and nurses sound medical. But it might be that the terms worry them and make them feel that the doctors are not telling them things they feel they ought to know.

In practice, this means that clinical staff should be clear about the need to engage people in language that they understand. One safe practice position might be simply to ensure that all communication is made in plain English, that complex terms are explained and a glossary of terms is published to make it easier for patients to understand what may have been said. It may also mean that practice staff routinely ask the following question: 'Sometimes we will use terms that you may not understand so is there anything anyone has said to you today that you are not clear about?'

How does the audience see us?

This is not always an easy question to answer, but it is important. We need to know what jumps into the head of the people to whom we send e-mails when they see that it is from us. This will make a difference to the way that our e-mail is read – or even if it is read at all. To some degree, how we are seen determines what action people take as a result of our communication.

In the busy world of primary care, finding out how our patients and partners see us could add an unmanageable layer of complexity to an already difficult situation. Patients have to be seen and time pressure already makes doing that challenging.

One quick way to understand how we are interpreted by our patients is to share information at practice meetings. Simply sharing information will give you personal feedback, in a non-threatening way, which will allow us to change the way we present ourselves in order to facilitate more effective communication.

Building up a picture of our audience

Some of the above points can be solved by asking the right questions of the right people. Undertake research and we will quickly be able to establish the way that a particular group of people sees the world.

Another technique is to create a visualisation of our audience. This is a technique whereby we put ourself, metaphorically, in the shoes of a particular member of our audience and try to see a situation as they would. In a clinical setting this can be particularly effective since we not only describe how the audience sees us but we can also start to mark out the emotional state that the audience may be in when encountering our practice.

Visualising is an exercise that can be done by groups of staff within the practice. It allows us both to examine how others might see our practice and to examine the assumptions that each member of staff is making about the people we deal with.

Here is an example of a business man who is anxious about his health.

The waiting room

I knew this was a mistake. A complete waste of time. I've stopped looking at my watch – it only makes me angry. A complete shambles from the word go – didn't have my name, wrong day, the consultant's not in today, just wait here for the moment. Moment – her word! And moment it most certainly is not. At least an hour so far.

It's probably all a fuss about nothing. But this fuss is costing me money. And the worst thing is I can't even use my mobile – something about interfering with medical equipment. As if. I haven't seen anyone do anything medical since I've been here.

If I was being charitable I'd be feeling grateful right now. I hate niggling pains. They eat away at your peace of mind. I feel drained by it. But these people are certainly not helping. Caring NHS. I don't think so.

Here they are again. More excuses. They might as well let me go. And I would walk out except I've waited six months already. Goodness knows how much longer I'd be left hanging on. It was a nightmare getting this far – Bob, my GP, helped pile the pressure on. He's as fed up with them as I am.

And this place is a tip. Stuff all over the place. If this was my office I'd be sacked. Chaos. The whole thing's like this – folk rushing about, a sense of panic. Nobody seems to know what anyone else is doing.

Makes you wonder where all the money goes. It's like hand-me-down city here. There are magazines that are about 10 years old, cracked plastic chairs, scuffed skirting boards. The shop has nothing in it. And the people behind the counter look as though they ought to be up in intensive care. If you don't feel ill when you come here you sure as hell will by the time you leave.

Maybe it's just me but you expect the caring professions to care, just a bit. I thought I'd count the number of people who looked in my direction and smiled but I had to abandon that – nobody even glanced my way. I read recently that these superbugs are hovering around hospitals so I'm keen to get out if I can. You read all the time that people go into hospital for little things – getting moles removed and that kind of thing – and then they never come out again. Or they do, but in a box.

The truth is that you're at their mercy. It's a bit like going to the garage with your car – they talk in code and then they're under the bonnet whipping things out and you haven't even said you want it done yet. Doctors are just the same. We kneel at their feet.

What's going on now – they're calling me. Typical: more of the same. They want me to go to another room about 40 miles from here. Have they got a map – no chance. Someone to go with me – some hope. No, it's just go and waste another hour of your life and wander aimlessly down some mile-long corridor and at least you'll be off our hands.

I don't know why I bothered. If I wasn't screaming in pain I wouldn't go near this place. And now I'm here it's making me feel worse.

How to use visualisation in a primary care setting

First, identify a member of the target audience. The stronger our initial understanding is, the more successful we are likely to be. Next, put ourself into the shoes of that person and into a situation where we might be trying to communicate with them. Then capture a moment in time. This could be the point at which this person approaches our reception or the point where they may have been given some bad news.

Write down exactly how we (as this person) see the situation in which we now find ourself. Do not edit it for style or effect. Rather, respond emotionally to the situation in as fulsome a way as possible. The purpose of the exercise is to gain an insight into our communication from another point of view.

Lastly, ensure that all members of staff are able to share each others' visualisations. Look for lessons that can be learned and use this information to alter the way in which we communicate with people from this audience in the future.

Key points

- Before you communicate with an audience on behalf of our practice, share as much information as possible.

- Be clear about whom we are communicating with.

- Understand the way in which they see the world.

- Understand and make use of the language that our audience will be comfortable with.

Channels

Channels are the means by which we get our message to the audiences we want to communicate with. We need to determine whether we will use them simply to supply information or whether we want feedback.

The channels we use should be determined largely by the ease with which our target audiences are able to access information. It would be relatively easy, for example, to make all our public information available on a practice website, but unless we were clear that everyone we were trying to reach had access to this facility, it would be a meaningless gesture.

We might want to know how many people have access to the internet. But, internet access will be just one of a number of barriers that will need to be considered when choosing our key channels.

Other questions include the following.

- *What are the levels of literacy among our target audience? Poor literacy is a key feature of British life today. It may be that as many as 15% of the people you want to reach with your messages will be unable to read them. This may mean choosing alternative, non-electronic channels for communication.*
- What channels do our target audience currently use?
- What are we competing with?

Messages

The idea behind messages or key messages is about simplifying what we say to our key audiences and repeating it over a period of time so that this produces desired actions or views. Key messages are likely to be common already in health as a means of persuading people to adopt a healthy lifestyle – 'Five a day' about eating fruit and vegetables, for example.

Essentially, we need to hone our messages so that they make sense to our key audiences. One way to achieve this quickly is to use some of the words that our audiences use.

Agree a small number of key messages

You may be tempted to have many messages, for many audiences. Broadly, given the level of communication that we are likely to undertake within our practice, the more messages you have, the less likely it is that they are going to have any real effect. For example, we may determine that we, as a practice, want to increase the number of people who have regular blood pressure checks. This is relatively easy to achieve with the patients we see because we can suggest this through practice nurses, in consultations and even through posters in the surgery.

But, by using patients as a communications medium, we may be able to create a key message that we say to each patient when they visit our practice, as a means of reaching their spouses, partners or other relatives. Our message may be simply: 'If you have a minute, ask your partner to pop in for a blood pressure check – undetected high blood pressure is one of the biggest killers in the country.'

If this message is repeated through all members of the practice to patients every time they visit, we will be able to evaluate its effectiveness by looking at the additional appointments made for blood pressure checks.

Key points

- Make our messages interesting and meaningful.
- Make our messages repeatable.
- Tie them to specific audiences.
- Tie them to key outcomes.
- Repeat them frequently and through a variety of channels.

Context

Remember that other things will shape how our communications will be interpreted. Our communications will not be the only thing that our target audience will be exposed to during the period that we are communicating with them. This is part of the problem. In all likelihood, we will be fighting for attention. And, if we are realistic, unless we are very skilled communicators, able to frame what we have to say in ways that make it clear to those with whom we communicate what the benefits are, we simply will not get through at all.

We should not be surprised by this. Yet, we assume, wrongly, that when we speak or write, others will hear, understand, assimilate and act on what we say. Begin by assuming that our communication will get no attention whatsoever and try to build from there.

However, it is worth going one step further. Even if our messages are getting through, there is no guarantee that they will be read in the way we might hope. The meaning of text depends very much upon the context around it. Take the following example.

> *We launched a campaign to promote health checks for men, and 40 men registered in the first week.*

Sounds like a good result?

> *The national average was 200 in similar practices.*

Looks like a failure now.

It is important that we are aware of the context within which our communications will be read. But in *political* organisations – in which individuals are interested in power and influence, and where 'small p' politics becomes one of the means by which people achieve their goals – other people will interpret or contextualise what we say and do.

If we accept this as a starting point (some people are uncomfortable with the idea that others will behave in untoward ways), it follows that we should know:

- who might recontextualise what we say
- how they will do it
- and with which audiences.

Another way to look at this is to consider who might gain by reinterpreting our message.

Of course, it is possible to become very conspiratorial about this very quickly, and to assume that others are out to reshape our messages. In most cases, our communication is barely on others' radar screens.

Evaluation

It is important to evaluate our communications. It takes time to plan and execute them so, as we have already learned, we should be clear about what we are trying to achieve before we set out. The review period is the means by which we establish whether or not our communication has worked.

We should try to evaluate communication activity in terms of the *outcome* we sought, rather than by the *output* we created. Inevitably, proper evaluation of communication is hard to achieve since there are many factors which affect the way that people behave. For this reason it is important that we set 'indicators', which will tell us whether things are working early on.

For example, we may establish an e-bulletin, which targets business people, offering advice on managing stress loads within a busy lifestyle. This could easily be written by medical staff and edited by a small primary care communications group. It could be dispatched on a monthly basis to people who have subscribed to it as a result of a blood pressure check at the practice. But, unless we have indicators that tell you that lifestyles have changed we might simply be sending out information that languishes in in-trays.

One way to approach this problem might be to build a small piece of research into your reception protocol so that repeat visitors who have received the e-bulletin are asked whether they have received the publication, whether they have used any information from it and whether they recall any of the items.

This approach, although not complex, can be an effective way of guiding our communication activity.

Similarly, if we use a strategic approach to manage our primary care e-mail practice, we might want to evaluate the impact that our new approach might have on key activities, such as the amount of time spent looking at e-mail, the negative impact that it has on effectiveness and so forth.

A final thought

One key part of the evaluation of an e-communications strategy is the ability to adjust our activity where our evaluation is showing us that the current approach is not working. If our strategy is no more than a document that the management team considers and notes, but never again reviews, we are likely to be wasting time, resources and energy:

> *'I see people do it all the time now. You'll be at a meeting and people will only be half there. They'll look as if they're listening but at every opportunity their heads will be down and they'll be looking at their Blackberries and they'll be e-mailing people. I was at a meeting seminar recently and I saw two managers e-mail each other during the session. The thing was they could have waited until after the session was finished and talked to each other. But they didn't. At the end, they went their separate ways. They didn't even look at each other.'*
>
> (Manager, talking about electronic communications)

e-Communicating

Mark Fletcher

'Then you should say what you mean,' the March Hare went on.
'I do,' Alice hastily replied; 'at least—at least I mean what I say—that's
the same thing, you know.'

'Not the same thing a bit!' said the Hatter. 'You might just as well say
that ''I see what I eat'' is the same thing as ''I eat what I see''!'
(Lewis Carroll, *Alice's Adventures in Wonderland*, 1865)

Electronic signature

The trouble with e-communication is that it is all over so quickly. E-mails appear disposable. We talk about dashing off e-mails as if we are making passing remarks in corridors. And that is the trouble: all the rules which apply to the rest of our communications, the stuff over which we will have sweated and fretted, apply to e-communications. But, more so.

The advent of the Blackberry and other electronic portable data assistants allows us to make every minute count. Where we might have passed the time of day with colleagues before meetings started, now we fire off a few missives electronically to people in other parts of the building. Often these are context-free – quick responses, single words, 'yes's' and 'no's'. Sometimes, we rant; our blood is up and we vent our anger on the way out to the car park.

And then, lo! All the things that we pride ourselves in – judgement, the careful balancing of opposing views, the ability to weigh up close but vaguely differentiable alternatives – vanish in an instant. The recipients will be the first to draw these obvious conclusions. But, in turn, others will, too. Because, just as we create e-mail quickly and without appropriate patience, so others forward it to yet more people. And the cycle of reputation decline goes on.

Before writing this chapter I read Mark Pallen's article 'Guide to the internet: electronic mail'.[1] Although it was published just a decade ago, it appeared to have been written in another era. Its detailed explanations of the constituent parts of electronic mail might now be more at home in a library on the ancient art of communication so familiar is the medium to the modern NHS.

And yet, whilst the idea of writing electronic mail is something few of us would flinch at, I am conscious that it is probably the most dangerous form of communication currently in existence. Few other means of getting our message across can, for most of us, have such massive potential implications. In the lifetime of the Blair government, at least two careers have ended because e-mails written at sensitive times were later quoted by the media. E-mails can become interesting currency.

When we communicate by e-mail we undertake many risks. Paradoxically, e-mail feels risk-free. How often we hear the words, 'I'll be with you in a minute, I'm just going to dash off a few e-mails.'

It is not uncommon for people to send e-mails during meetings. The arrival of the Blackberry means that many of us are able to send e-mails whilst on the train, over breakfast and doubtless some e-obsessed individuals send them from the bath.

We treat e-mail as we would conversation. Typically, our electronic messages are occasionally spiced with jokes and untoward comments. Without wishing to spoil the fun, this chapter has been written to try to tease out some lessons for writing effective e-mails and being able to weigh up the risks of doing otherwise.

Writing electronically is different from other forms of communication. E-mail may be the fastest way to get our message to an individual but it may languish in their in-box for months. Or, worse, it may be deleted immediately. And even if someone opens our e-mail, there is no guarantee that they will give it sufficient attention to make sense of it.

E-writing is a relatively new form of communication. We tend to treat e-mail in one of two ways – either as letters by another means or as conversation. In reality, it is neither. Letters tend to be linear in construction. We set out at the top of a letter the purpose of the communication. This will often be followed by an explanation of the letter itself, which culminates in our request or comment. In other words, we outline, contextualise and then communicate.

Conversation is quite different. In a conversation two or more individuals share the context. But this may never be written down. Rather, a shared understanding of the nature of the communication will enable the participating individuals to make comments which, viewed separately, may be perceived to be either meaningless or to convey the opposite of that which is understood by the participants.

In e-mail, we are conscious that individuals have little attention. So we often feel the need to get to the point quickly. And therein lies the challenge: how do we balance the need to contextualise the request at the same time as needing to hold the attention of the recipient. This chapter looks at how we can increase the effectiveness of our electronic communications.

The critical data

When an e-mail arrives in our in-box, our decision to open it, ignore it or delete it will be based upon how we view certain key data.

- Who sent it?
- What does the header say?
- Is it easy to grasp in one look?
- Is it easy to deal with now?
- What will happen if I ignore it?

Who sent me this?

Some people's e-mails are never ignored. Broadly, these are influential or important people who matter in your working life. There will be a similar group of people in our personal life. We read their e-mails either because we feel we have to or because we feel we need to.

The recipients of our e-mails will make similar judgements about us. If we are to increase the effectiveness of our electronic communications, we need to understand the associations that will jump into the minds of the people to whom we send e-mail when something arrives from us. In other words, what do *we* mean to people?

This information, although crucial for day-to-day communication, is not the easiest to collect. In reality, most of us never ask the question, 'How do you see me?' This is mainly because the response is either dishonest – people will not seek to hurt us by telling the truth and we will therefore learn nothing – or it may be honest, in which case we may hear things we would really rather not.

But, it is vital that we know. In the worst-case scenario, we may be sending e-mail that is never read simply because people find our communication dull, uninteresting and ignorable. Yet, our communication may affect clinical outcomes.

Finding out what people think

One way of gathering this information is to gather it consciously but discreetly. It is possible to assemble a clear picture of how we and our colleagues are viewed by the people with whom we communicate regularly. In practice, it is difficult to find out what everyone thinks of us. So, first, we must prioritise.

This means determining who really matters to our team or practice. Then we can systematically set about finding out how those people see us and our colleagues. Most of this work will have to be done covertly. In a sensitive environment it can be difficult to undertake systematic formal research. Doing so in this area would inevitably raise questions about why we might be asking the questions. Also, given the nature of the material we are likely to uncover between the lines, honesty may evaporate as formality increases.

Below are some questions to think about.

Do they know who we are?

It is relatively easy to assume that others know who we are. In reality, we may not even exist in their lives.

What do they associate with us?

This may be no more than, 'Oh, she's that doctor from Blankley Medical Centre.' Or it may be that we are associated with a key project. Or, worse, it may be that the only time we appeared on the horizon we were part of some problem, 'Not him again – every time I hear from him it's a problem.'

What words jump to mind when they read, see or hear our name?

This is critical data since it is likely that those same words will appear as our e-mail pops into their in-box. This data will have to be pieced together from passing remarks and from inference. We and our colleagues will hear things said about us and our team members from time to time. The key is to assemble this information and share it.

How believable or credible are we?

Here, we are looking for an indicator of reliability or trust. The more credible we are, the more we will be trusted.

How useful are we perceived to be?

The assumption under this question is simple: the more we are able to help others achieve what they are trying to achieve, the more likely they are to view our communications positively.

What is our 'brand'?

The hardest question of all, since what it refers to is an understanding of how others perceive what we are about. Again, we are looking for a word or phrase that captures how others see us. We may be a nurse practitioner by job title, but certain key individuals might perceive us as a 'heavyweight' or a key influencer of other important people.

In one sense, the above information is absolutely critical. The remainder of this chapter is concerned with how to maximise the attention that our electronic communication will get. But, if our e-mail is not perceived to be important simply because we are not important either, it is questionable whether anything else we write will be read. If that is the case, the solution lies not in improving our communication techniques but in changing the nature of our reputation.

The header

After a recipient has established that our e-mail might be worth reading they will quickly turn their attention to the header line. In just a few words, we can grab attention or we can condemn our e-mail to the 'Deleted' box for ever. The core question that should be in our mind before we even think about writing the header is this: 'What's in my communication that will benefit the recipient?'

All too often, we concern ourselves with matters that affect *us*. In all honesty, we select communications that benefit us directly – though we may wrap our selection up in all sorts of complex rationales. Turn this on its head and we will find very quickly that the more we are able to turn the header into the solution to our recipient's problems, the more attention we are likely to get.

Because it is composed of few words, the header is also the place where our verbosity and lack of focus will be confirmed, although, in fairness, it may be hard to prove that we are not really worth reading until the end of the first sentence.

So there are some things to think about before writing the header.

- What are the potential benefits of my e-mail to the recipient?
- How can I frame that in no more than six to ten words?
- Which key words will instantly get his or her attention?
- How can I capture the essence of what I want quickly?

This could turn the following header:

> *Practice meeting 3 pm – agenda attached*

into:

> *Meeting at 3 to resolve staff rotas*

or:

> *Staff rotas part 2 – your wisdom needed at 3 pm*

Although the latter two are less formal and, it could be argued, more flippant – particularly given the serious nature of the discussion on staff rotas, which are only displaced in importance by staff car parking – the justification is in the outcome. People will read our e-mail and act as we want them to.

The body copy

Because it is one-to-one communication (otherwise it is spam), e-mail demands more of us as writers. Imagine we were briefing a colleague on a difficult piece of work. To ensure that they had the time to listen and assimilate what we were going to say to them, we might suggest that we both set aside half an hour at the end of the day to discuss things. We would doubtless make this suggestion early on to enable our colleague to shift their diary. And we would check as the day progressed that their priorities had not shifted. When you reached the allotted time, we would know that, barring interruptions, we would get their undivided attention.

What we would not do is stop our colleague in the corridor and launch into 600 words of text – three minutes of non-stop speaking – as a way of taking the issue forward. If, because of the pressure of work, we were forced to brief our colleague very quickly, we would introduce it with a warning, 'Sorry Bob, I'm going to have to bring you up to date on something which could go pear-shaped today, have you got a minute?'

Not doing so would quickly cause our colleagues to assume that we had few social skills and that we missed out on the tact and diplomacy modules at school. Yet, how many e-mails make exactly the same demands upon our attention. They appear in the in-box and when you click them open they hit you between the eyes with pages of text which, unless they involve the loss or potential loss of life, we ignore.

Here are some tips to make sure that people read the body text in our e-mails.

Set out the implications at the start of the e-mail

It will help our reader if they understand immediately what this communication might mean:

> *This short note is designed to bring you up to date on the staff car parking. It's to be discussed this afternoon at three. It's important that you read it because I suspect that staff will be upset if we implement the practice policy.*

Say what you expect the recipient to do

Our note could be for information, for background or for action:

> *I'd like you to take a look at the attached file and let me know what you think by 2.30. If you are not going to have time to read it please let me know by 1.30. Otherwise I'll assume that you're conversant with all of the arguments.*

Sort out what we are going to say, and the outcome we want, before we put fingers to the keyboard

Do not start writing immediately. There is something about taking action that feels reassuring to us. This can be fine for day-to-day e-mails when we are doing nothing complex. But, since we increasingly rely on e-mail as our main channel of communication, it is likely that some of the emotions that would have been reserved only for ranting sessions in the corridor will now turn up in our electronic exchanges. And just as we would probably have had time to cool down in the car park before we told our colleagues how stupid their ideas are, so we need to afford ourselves the same breathing space in e-mail. Don't do this kind of thing:

> *John, Maureen has just passed me your note and I actually don't understand what you're playing at on this issue – staff will be upset – and it's typical of the way you are approaching things in general at the moment.*

Remember that e-mail is currency

Every single one of us will have e-mails that have been passed to us by others who are keen to demonstrate the errant ways of our colleagues, 'I thought you'd like to see the kind of thing I have to put up with.' e-Mails are not only currency today and affect how we might see a particular individual; they are also historical reference points. Anything that appears in the body copy of one e-mail could turn into the bcc version to another person.

Say what we can, if possible, in a single-screen grab

It is not always possible to condense our communication into a few short sentences. But it often is. The trouble is that – and this situation is made worse by personal data assistants – we tend to write as we think. Crucially, we must get to the point quickly. It means putting the key information at the top of the e-mail. It means abandoning the established practice of putting all the context in place before we make our point.

Use a good mix of short and longer sentences

Look at the BBC website for examples of excellent e-writing. On the news front page you will find headlines in five to seven words and sentences in 20–25 words. Apart from knowing that much of their content will be either originated or edited by journalists, e-writers know that readers like to get to the facts quickly. It is also far easier for the eye to grab at a single look. The rhythm of a well-crafted piece of text will instantly make us more readable. Look at the following:

> *This e-mail will bring you up to date on some of the developments of the staff car parking policy which you will be aware has been rumbling on for ages now – I think Toby's paper is worth reading, he circulated it last week – do you have a copy? Let me know if not and I'll send one over. We want to meet later to discuss this at around three-ish if you're free – if not could you let my PA know. I'd like to sort this thing out today if possible. Anyway, let me know what you think. (97 words)*

> *We're meeting at three to sort out staff car parking. Please read Toby's paper. If you want a copy let me know. If you can't make it, call Trish. (29 words)*

Hone our communication for the audience

Literally, build a message that delivers the outcome we want. This means finding the right words that say the right things to this person. Curiously, forwarded e-mails make this all the harder since an e-mail written for one audience will potentially mean quite different things to different audiences.

Developing an e-communications policy

No communication is risk-free. The way that our communication will be read, understood or acted upon will be a product of many factors, some of which will be beyond our control. However, where a passing remark may precipitate an untoward reaction of behaviour, other than through the recollections of the receiver and other accounts (hearsay, witnesses or sup-position), it will only exist in the memories of one of two people. E-mail is different. A comment made in haste will live in others' in-boxes and on the server for ever (depending on your practice policy). It will be searchable, copy-able and capable of being endlessly reproduced with no loss of quality. Furthermore, if it refers to a patient it may be requested and scrutinised by that person and viewed in an altogether different light. e-Communication is a potential source of risk to our practice.

One way of reducing or at least quantifying risk is to develop a policy that governs our use of electronic communication. All too often we assume that everyone has the right to communicate by e-mail without fear or fetter. Given the potential consequences of such an approach, there are merits in being clear about who should be able to send messages to different people.

In what circumstances should you send e-mail?

e-Mail, as has already been acknowledged, is not a flawless form of communication. The danger is that we send e-mail because it is easy and apparently quick. But, looked at from the point of view of the recipient, the fact that we send e-mail rather than write formally or speak face to face might cause others to see us in a negative light.

Given the way that others will read our acts as intentional (even where they may be less considered), we should seek to adopt a consistent practice policy that specifies the circumstances in which we should send e-mail. It may be that we use e-mail in many circumstances simply to confirm a face-to-face discussion and agreement. In which case we might sign off our e-mail with a request that the recipient both confirm receipt and agree our understanding or otherwise. Our policy may include:

- confirmation of the outcomes of face-to-face discussions
- requests for information
- details of appointments
- clinical data sent to other primary and secondary care colleagues.

It is possible for e-mail to bring an organisation into disrepute. Electronic communication can be used to send everything from humour to malicious gossip. These, and other forms of communication, could present challenges to our practice reputation and should be specified within the policy. Obvious as this may sound, unless it is written down and agreed, it is possible for colleagues to argue that there is 'no harm in occasional humour'. In the most innocent sets of circumstances this may be true. But, viewed through the lens of the worst-case scenario, we may see it differently.

To whom should it be sent?

In local health economies, it is often possible to have access to the addresses of a wide range of people. Global e-mails and communication that is sent indiscriminately to groups of people without rationale or reason can cause recipients to view all our communications negatively. One way to avoid this to agree the circumstances in which key people – those whose views about you could shape your career, success or failure – will be written to. This can be reviewed by the whole team on a regular basis.

Reference

1   Pallen M (1995) Guide to the internet: electronic mail. *BMJ* **311**: 1487–90.

11

The peculiarity of e-communication

Mark Fletcher

Go to any meeting involving any senior people in the public sector these days and we will be bewildered by technology. Everyone, it seems, is becoming addicted to maximum availability. It will not be uncommon to watch people texting or e-mailing during meetings. This short chapter is a reflection on some of the issues arising from the use of 'always on' thinking.

It's all on the record

Unlike conversation, which relies on a third party to report our exchanges for the record, e-communication is entirely visible. Everything we have ever written could be stored somewhere. This includes everything from carefully crafted missives to thumb-typed sharp notes fired off in the heat of the moment between or even during meetings.

Furthermore, anything we write can and may be used in evidence against us at some stage. If this sounds a bit negative, ask ourselves how many times we have been copied into someone else's exchanges so that we can marvel at the sensitivity of their language and expression.

e-Games are entirely acceptable

e-Mail is set up to enable us to do things that we might otherwise think underhand. Carbon copying, blind carbon copying and forwarding appear to be quite normal activities. In reality, it is likely that a good deal of the mail we choose to share with others is sent for other than the best possible reasons.

Carbon copying

Simply copying people into exchanges where all parties can see the communication can be helpful. But are our additional recipients clear about why they are being shown the material? Frequently, we will talk about ensuring that others are 'kept in the loop'. Broadly, though, a good deal of communication is carbon copied as an insurance policy, protecting us if the worst occurs. In such circumstances, doubtless we will point to the many relevant e-mails and proclaim our innocence, saying that our managers or superiors were entirely cognisant of this business.

There are merits in identifying the circumstances in which carbon copying may be acceptable in our e-communications policy. Specifically, we may wish to consider what the implications are for the recipient. If it is our practice policy to ensure that our practice manager is copied in, for example, on all sensitive communications then we should be clear about what we expect this person to do about it.

- Should such communication simply be noted?
- Should it be brought forward to regular meetings for consideration or review?
- Should the practice manager comment on the exchanges?
- Do we anticipate circumstances in which the practice manager may need to adduce this as evidence on sensitive matters?

All in all, we probably copy people into exchanges intermittently. Or where we feel particularly exposed on an issue. Or to demonstrate that we are acting as others anticipate we should. But, given the sensitivity around e-communication, in particular, given the demands of the Freedom of Information Act, this may be a matter to consider.

Blind carbon copying

This is another matter altogether. The ease with which we are now able to do this should not mask the nature of the act itself. To put it in context, imagine that every time we wanted to blind carbon copy, we had to take the piece of correspondence to the photocopier where you are likely to meet other people. If, when we are asked the question, 'What are you copying?', we feel a twinge of embarrassment, we realise that we are engaged in a devious act.

The essence of blind carbon copying is to enable a third party to make a judgement about an exchange without the knowledge of the person with whom we are communicating. This might seem entirely reasonable until we consider that if we are doing this regularly, the chances are that every other person with whom we are communicating is likely to be doing the same.

The implications of this are that we should begin by assuming that every e-exchange is being considered by others all the time. It is unlikely to be so. But since we cannot tell what has been blind carbon copied, it is best to assume that virtually all communication that could have a negative impact on us or our organisation's reputation could fall into this category.

Forwarding exchanges

Broadly, we forward entire exchanges to others to make a point or to enable them to make a judgement. Read back through your e-mail files and, where you have forwarded exchanges to others, check whether you have copied this for information to the person with whom you have had the original correspondence. If not, it is likely you had some motive in not doing so.

All these practices, while common enough, increase risk around our communications. Risk here is defined as activity which could affect the way in which us or our organisation is seen or trusted by key audiences. This chapter is not suggesting that we should not undertake such practices: doing so is neither likely nor possible. We all engage in other, similar activities in our day-to-day communication – gossip, passing on exchanges to others, equivocation, reinterpretation. But, because of the peculiarity of e-communication, the fact that it is all on the record – it is better to do such things wittingly and fully aware of the risk.

Managing e-risk

Just to be clear: risk, in this context, is about activity that could affect the way in which we or our organisation is seen or trusted by key audiences. By implication, we need to know who our key audiences are, and on what basis they trust us. e-Communication is highly portable. An exchange between colleagues in a trust could easily find its way in to the in-box of our local MP or even into a ministerial box.

As a practice, map out the key audiences upon whose support we depend. To look at this another way, who are the people without whose support we could not continue to work?

Other ways of assessing communication risk

What is the worst that could happen?

In practical terms, it can be hard to weigh up the risk on every single piece of e-mail. But, given the potential damage that a single untoward exchange could cause, it is worth considering this question every time we send an e-mail. That is not to say that we should abandon all e-communication. Rather, we should take account of risk wittingly.

Is it likely?

There is a danger of many things; the question of likelihood is another matter. Think about the factors that could make the worst case more, rather than less, likely. There may be individuals or interests – think about the local media – who will make it their business to ask legitimate questions and seek access to exchanges on sensitive matters.

What is my fallback position?

If the worst should happen, what will we do? Are we prepared? We have fire doors and extinguishers because fires are always possible. Do we have a similar practice position should an untoward exchange find itself being quoted by a local MP in the newspaper? The time to worry about our fallback position is not when it is needed. Preparation is the key to protecting our reputation.

How can we mitigate the risk?

Blind carbon copying and letting others 'in on the secret' are some of the ways in which we mitigate risk. Our assumption is often based on the idea that if someone else, particularly in a position of power, knows about an exchange, we are somehow protected. If this is one of the ways in which we mitigate risk it is worth checking this with those to whom we copy our correspondence. They might see this quite differently and, in the worst case, might, not unreasonably, leave us to stew in our own juice. Again, do not wait for this to happen before discovering that we are on our own.

Can we achieve a similar or better outcome by another means?

One way to reduce some of the risk arising from e-communication is to use other channels. A great deal can be achieved by picking up the telephone or by arranging meetings. It is not always so quick and we cannot use a Blackberry or a hand-held computer, but it can make things a lot better in the worst case.

Part 4: Resource pack

12

Case study 1: People with sight loss, of South Asian origin, in Bradford

Mark Gibson and Pam Turpin

Introduction

Preliminary qualitative data collection carried out as part of the Medicines Information Needs for Older People with Sight Loss (MINOPS) project* reveal that, in Bradford, older people with a disability such as sight loss find that a lot of healthcare services are largely inaccessible to them. Some of those interviewed for the project were not only older with sight loss, but they were also from South Asian communities and spoke a first language other than English. Furthermore, they received multiple medications for more than one chronic disease on a regular, repeat basis and were regular visitors to their GPs' surgeries. The opinions raised by these participants are

*The Medicines Information Needs for Older People with Sight Loss (MINOPS) is a project based at the University of Leeds, which receives funding from the Community Fund via the Royal National Institute of the Blind (RNIB). The research aims to find out what medicine information that older people with sight loss need, to describe whether there are any gaps in how information is provided and how this situation can be improved. The study is being conducted in the Bradford area which, based on the city's demographic composition, focuses on elderly people with visual disability, as well as low income and unemployed households, people from South Asian communities and those with a limited knowledge of English. For more information about this project, please contact Mark Gibson (m.j.gibson@leeds.ac.uk).

based on their own experiences and frequently identify various facets of doctor–patient communication as a major area for concern and source of potential exclusion.

The evidence

One person asserted that people who speak a language other than English are, to a certain extent, socially disabled in the UK. Sometimes their patient confidentiality is compromised, such as when older people have to bring a younger relative (perhaps a daughter or a sister) to the GP's surgery, to deal with potentially embarrassing conditions such as gynaecological complaints. Not only could this be regarded as an invasion of privacy and dignity for the patient, it is also recognised as a difficult situation for both the GP and the younger relative, because much of the GP's message may be lost, as many younger people would not appreciate the medical terminology in either language.

To avoid these situations, it was suggested that both patients and GPs need to be able to anticipate the consultation, and make arrangements in advance to provide multilingual assistance. This help could come in the form of interpreters or liaison workers, as well as through written and audio information.

To achieve this, GPs need to record details about their patients alongside other information such as address and religion, for example. One participant who had taught himself IT skills in older age suggested a possible way for GPs to record information about individual patients:

> 'It could be difficult for GPs and other healthcare staff to identify which languages people speak, and require information in, but it would be quite simple for GPs to have a box within the patient record on the computer which would enable them to record this kind of information as well as other individual information needs, for example "Patient does not speak English. He/she requires an interpreter in 'X' language." Or "Patient is visually impaired", "Prefers information sent to him/her in such-and-such a format". It's not difficult to make these adjustments on the records. So, as soon as a person makes an appointment, the doctor can access this information in advance of the consultation and can look after individual needs this way. It's just an extra field in a database.'

Other reported problems relating to clinician–patient communication concerned medicines information, namely, why patients need to adhere to a given course of treatment. One older male participant reported that many people of South Asian origin do not take their prescribed high blood pressure medications:

'They are reluctant to take these medications because they think if they have this disease already, there's nothing they can do and no medication will make it better. The fact is taking the medication does help and you have to come to terms with it. Maybe you just need a bit more encouragement from the GP or the nurse, but this is not often forthcoming. So, the onus is not just on the individual but also on those involved in the provision of healthcare, as well as the carers. If the patient does not take the medication correctly and on time, then obviously this is going to cost the NHS much more later on.'

However, communication is not always concerned with a person's medical needs. For people with disabilities, for instance, GPs' surgeries could send messages based on how physically accessible their buildings are and what processes are in place in the reception area to cater for people with particular needs. One participant explained:

'The medical centre I attend has colour-coded queues, electronic information boards where the names of the doctors appear, along with the name of the next patient in the queue. I complained to the practice manager that this is not appropriate, not just for visually impaired and blind people, but for people who have problems with reading. You just don't know when it's your turn and unless you have a white stick to denote that you are blind, nobody will come to help, nobody will even know you need help. Now, my doctor always comes out when he calls me in. I think the practice manager must have put a special note on the computer to notify the doctor of my needs. So, once I manage to access the doctor, I find communication is very good.'

Electronic information boards, therefore, are one application of technology in general practice which is unhelpful and problematic for patients. Another participant also touched upon this subject and suggested:

'There are many simple solutions for GP surgeries to be more inclusive for people with sight loss. For example, instead of flashing lights on overhead electronic display screens, GPs could announce their next patient over a tannoy system, which is bound to be cheaper for them. Many practices place barriers in the way of people and we keep having to rely on other people to help us achieve very simple goals – such as visiting your GP.'

Although still at an exploratory stage, it is clear that for the participants recruited as part of the MINOPS study, being older, having sight loss and maybe more than one chronic illness, speaking a first language that is not English is simply one more dimension to the kind of exclusion perceived as preventing them from receiving the care they believe they are entitled to from primary care services.

Discussion

This short chapter has examined societal multilingualism in a UK context, and has painted a picture of a very complex, and often underappreciated, aspect of life in the UK. Various health inequalities were identified among speakers of languages other than English, as well as people who belong to the black and ethnic minority communities in the UK. A number of IT applications were presented: these aim to provide multilingual health information for both patients and professionals involved in primary care. Finally, a selection of qualitative data collected during the initial stages of the MINOPS project was introduced to highlight ways in which, according to the participants in the study, doctor–patient communication improved and health inequalities can alleviated be in some way.

13

Case study 2: The secondary care perspective

Charlotte Bates

In France it is rude to let a conversation drop; in England it is rash to keep it up. No one there will blame you for silence. When you have not opened your mouth for three years, they will think, 'This Frenchman is a nice quiet fellow.'

(André Maurois, *Three Letters on the English*)[1]

Setting the scene

Accident & Emergency (A&E) departments are hubs of hospital activity. Busy round the clock, a high throughput of patients and staff: critical decisions are made with and about patients under the widest variety of circumstances. Good communication is vital in A&E – from face-to-face communication between staff and patients to the more subtle influences exerted over our daily practice by external agencies.

This chapter explores the issues and lines of communication (Figure 13.1) between A&E, the patient and medical colleagues working in primary care. The aim is to illuminate what happens now – if we understand it, we can work with it – but also to diagnose where some of the pitfalls might be found and to offer some dynamic changes for the future benefit of our shared goal: the patient's health and well-being (Figure 13.2).

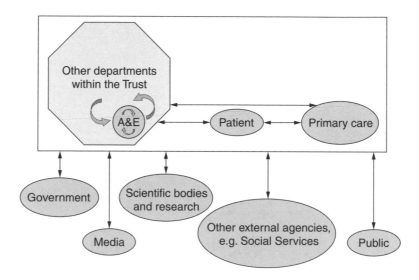

Figure 13.1 Lines of communication.

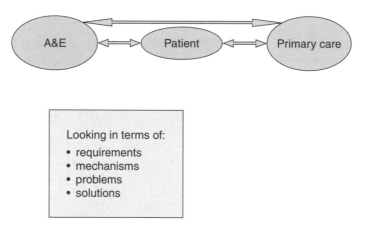

Figure 13.2 The focus for analysis.

Communications requirements

Teams in A&E require more and more information from patients and the community in order to do the job of patient care. The availability of the correct information is vital to efficient practice and no one would dispute that an informed decision is usually best.

Communication on an individual level

Patients may turn up at A&E by themselves, or be sent directly or indirectly by primary care providers. On an individual level, communication usually starts when the patient arrives at the reception desk. The patient will be asked questions to obtain their demographic details and to elicit information about their complaint. Patients may have been seen by their GP before their visit to A&E. For the A&E team, any information about the patient's complaint, details of any investigations done and advice and treatment given is invaluable. It permits fast-tracking of the patient within the department and can speed up the whole process, improving the patient's experience, due to a simple bit of communication between colleagues. Equally, after patients have attended A&E it is essential that we have an efficient and foolproof way of communicating back to primary care any important investigations or diagnoses made, in order to avoid duplication of effort and confusion. Doctors and nurses working in the patient's own general practice need to be aware of what advice has been given and what follow-up is necessary to ensure consistency and a seamless progression of care.

It is often the case that results and reports are available only after a patient has been discharged home. In some cases these reports or results might differ from what was thought to be the case during the A&E attendance – some things simply show up after the fact. It is vitally important that this type of information is communicated to primary care teams (and, if necessary, directly to the patient) along with appropriate instructions about any further action that may be required.

Sometimes it is necessary to have prior notice of problems or to set management plans for certain patients if their attendance is unpredictable. This may be because a patient is known to be violent towards healthcare workers or because the patient has some ongoing health issues that are best dealt with in a planned manner. If there are problems that have become apparent only during a patient's management within secondary care facilities, these and their management plans need to be communicated back to the primary care givers and other A&E departments.

Interdepartmental communication

As primary care and A&E staff work in very similar spheres it is imperative that both are made aware of any important policy changes within either system. It is also valuable to know of any referral pathways available within the local primary care system in order to direct patients to the fastest and most appropriate means of referral. Ideally, this arrangement would be reciprocal and GPs should be made aware of any new care pathways in use and any limitations in the referral pathways available in A&E.

In these days of ongoing appraisal and evidence-based medicine it is important that teams in A&E and in primary care talk to each other about training needs and courses available for staff. There is a lot of common ground here and the overlap in training requirements, pooling of resources and utilization of the wide knowledge base available in both A&E and primary care offers a win–win situation. Good relationships are key to good practice, and learning together might be a new and innovative way of not only seeing the scenery from a different window, but of forging contacts and relationships which can be the essential framework of good communications.

Often, when the patient leaves the department, the A&E team receives little feedback about problems or successes. It is the primary care teams which are privy to that story. They say that 'If you always do what you always did, you will always get what you always got'. From a risk management point of view, some way of sharing informal feedback between primary care and A&E teams about problems or successes would be appreciated and valuable in the constant efforts to improve practice and the patient experience. Of course there must also be a formal but user-friendly system in place for complaints, which allows speedy action to be taken to avoid further problems and build on past successes. But some other way of sharing the good and bad parts of the patient's experience must be another communication avenue that primary care and A&E teams should explore together.

Communications: some problems and some solutions

Face-to-face communication: keeping the secrets secret

Most communication involving patients directly is face to face: between the patient and primary care team and between the patient and A&E staff. There are inherent difficulties with the face-to-face experience. Perhaps the most obvious is the provision of adequate privacy to ensure patient confidentiality; the age-old problem of patient details being ascertained over a relatively open desk in the reception areas of both general practice surgeries and A&E departments. Some of these problems can be overcome by minimising the amount of information that is obtained in this manner. Computerised systems have improved this interface with the patient with their ability to draw upon information that is already known about the patient once the basic demographics are ascertained. The efficiency of these systems would be improved further if primary care and A&E could share access to a core spine of patient information. The situation should improve with the introduction of primary care staff 'out of hours' into A&E departments.

Face-to-face communication: informed consent

Patient competency is also an important issue here. The unconscious patient's lack of competency is usually self-evident, however, in patients with reduced mental capacity it may be less obvious and may be overlooked. Again, shared access to the wealth of computerised patient information already stored would be invaluable in these situations.

Face-to-face communication: language as a barrier

Occasionally a language or cultural barrier causes difficulties in the face-to-face patient experience. If available, the best solution in these circumstances is using the language skills of on-site staff. However, often family members or local interpreters have to be relied upon, whether in person or even by telephone. The use of family members or local interpreters engenders further problems of patient confidentiality and the effect of receiving information about the details of medical complaints second hand. Problems to do with cultural barriers are perhaps best dealt with by training. Staff need a basic knowledge of the local different cultures and an understanding of the sensitivity which needs to be displayed when interacting with patients. As already explained, there can be problems when information, in particular medical information, is relayed via a third party, and this indirect spread of information can sometimes be detrimental to face-to-face communication with the patient.

Face-to-face communication: teamwork

Face-to-face communication also occurs directly between A&E and primary care teams, sometimes in the form of planned meetings to discuss new policies, care pathways or specific patients, and sometimes more informally through chance meetings. These chance meetings may become more commonplace with the introduction of primary care staff into A&E departments for the new ways of working the 'out of hours' service. This direct communication between primary care and A&E creates problems of ensuring the adequate documentation of information exchanged at a chance meeting and the dissemination of information discussed at formal meetings. Putting minutes of meetings into electronic form to be accessible to all concerned is one solution to the dissemination issue but it is difficult to ensure adequate documentation of communication through more informal meetings.

Written communication

The vast quantities of paperwork generated by A&E departments and the primary care sector threatens the forests of the world but provides a huge proportion of information available to both. It encompasses everything, from casualty cards and GP patient Lloyd-George records to flyers for various meetings, and a mountain of journals, reports and policy. Even Post-it messages left between staff create their own problems, but provide a backbone of communications between teams working different shifts and running between care settings.

Patient confidentiality must be paramount and may be breached if paperwork is not strictly policed or is left lying about for others to view. This is often a particular problem in an A&E department where departmental layouts, numerous staff and attendance of other specialities all contribute to the problem. Post-it notes can provide a source of inadvertent breaches of confidentiality and should be discouraged for all but the most basic and impersonal messages, especially bearing in mind that such messages often go missing and may not be passed on.

Missing paperwork is the source of much anxiety both for current problems, for example when responding to telephone enquiries about the progress of patients, or when records need to be consulted retrospectively when complaints are received. Not only is there the possibility of paperwork being lost within the various departments but also when information is transferred in this manner between A&E, the patient and the GP practice. At present we rely on both internal and external postal systems, with their own inherent problems. To minimise the problem of missing paperwork we should, first, work to reduce the volume of paperwork generated by avoiding duplication and, second, have robust filing systems and procedures in place which all staff must comply with when handling the various forms of paperwork used. Some A&E departments and GP practices are investigating the possibility of a 'paper-free' environment. This is a solution that has been used to good effect in the USA and perhaps we should learn from their experience.

Telecommunications

The telephone is a much used and abused means of communication in both A&E and primary care. There are similar problems here with face-to-face communication: lack of documentation and reliable recording of conversations, messages being relayed by third parties and issues of confidentiality raised by conversations being overheard. Answerphones provide yet further possible problems of confidentiality and a potential breakdown in communication if messages are left on the wrong answerphone or picked up by the wrong recipient. Again, some of these problems may be addressed by minimising the use of the telephone as a means of communication. Some of the documentation issues have been dealt with by the introduction of NHS Direct, where most patient advice calls are now directed. With the inherent dangers of leaving messages on answerphones it would seem wise that a policy of never using answerphones should be in place for all health workers; however, in the primary care sector this will not always be practicable.

It should always be remembered that, with certain vulnerable patients, a telephone call as a means of communication can be a frightening and confusing experience, and in such circumstances planning the communication in advance can prove helpful.

A common practice in most A&E departments is to obtain patient medication lists from GP surgeries by telephone. Sometimes there may be confusion with similar-sounding medications and even if this is avoided by spelling certain words this can be a very time-consuming process for A&E and primary care staff alike. The obvious solution here is, again, shared access to important patient information, for example a recent medication list. The other advantage of having this information available in a computerised form would be that it could be accessed out of hours.

A more recent application of telecommunications has been the possibility of digital images of certain complaints and injuries being communicated between specialities and, indeed, between primary and secondary caregivers when advice is sought. As all digital images constitute data, this raises the possibility of consent and data protection issues in the future.

A perhaps not insignificant consideration with telecommunications is cost, especially following the ever-increasing popularity of mobile phones. If carrying mobile phones for the purposes of sending digital images becomes commonplace it is easy to see that the telecommunications costs would be considerably increased. Perhaps, in the future, patients will be requested to provide not only their telephone contact details but also an e-mail address, if available.

Photocopying and facsimile

Many A&E departments rely on carbon copies of patients' notes to provide the communication link back to the GP and primary care team. Quite apart from the difficulties engendered when trying to decipher other people's handwriting, there may also be problems with the quality of print after the carbon-copying process. This problem of print quality will be magnified following the government directive in England that all communication between the hospital doctor and the GP be copied to the patient. Often, different colours of paper are used to indicate the different uses of these copies, this can lead to further problems if these copies are then photocopied as certain colours of paper do not photocopy well. Only using the photo-copying facility for printed documents could eliminate handwriting and copy quality difficulties; however, at present this is probably not practicable in most departments.

Similar problems are encountered when information is faxed to the recipient. There is also the problem peculiar to faxing of there being very little control over where the information is sent to and mistakes with wrong numbers are reasonably commonplace. This causes a potential risk and possible difficulties proving that information was either sent or received, should the need arise, unless a documented faxed date facility is available. For these reasons facsimiles should rarely be used as a form of communi-cation for important or sensitive information and, if used at all, a telephone call should also be made to confirm the arrival of the correct information with the recipient.

Computer systems and e-communication

Many of the problems already highlighted by the other forms of communi-cation in use at present could be solved by the introduction of a compre-hensive computerised system with dual access by A&E and primary care. In an ideal world, all patient interaction could be recorded electronically from attendances to investigations, results, diagnoses and follow-up plans.

Primary care has probably made further advances in this field than A&E. Most GPs are now using computers during the consultation process, to say nothing of computer use in the practice management arena. The majority of general practice surgeries seem to be moving towards varying degrees of paper-light environments.

Some A&E departments are rising to the challenge with some already sending discharge information to primary caregivers via e-mail, utilising the automatic reply systems to ensure their arrival at their intended destin-ation. Nearly all A&E departments now have some form of computerised communication system with some of the more innovative having all investigations and results accessible via computer. Several departments have even started to consider the possibility of entering details of the patient consultation and examination directly in computers with the possibility of hand-held modules coming into play. The natural progression would be to combine all this information held by GPs and A&E on one central system accessible by both.

Although a lot of the problems of handwriting, lost documentation and dissemination might be alleviated by such computerised systems the issues of confidentiality and patient competency remain. There is also a new set of problems, including staff training, the danger of less information being documented as people find typing more time-consuming and difficulty with drawings and diagrammatic notation. Of course, the initial cost of such systems can be staggering and other disadvantages of the paper-free system are the possibility of system failure or access being gained by inappropriate persons. The only solutions are extremely robust back-up systems and comprehensive and constantly updated security software.

Final thoughts

The amount of information required to be communicated between A&E, the patient and primary care is huge and varied, but the aim is the same – to hit the quality care goal. At present the mechanisms by which this goal is achieved are also many and varied. The current state of affairs leads to a host of problems and is extremely difficult to police. Although by no means eliminating all these problems, it does appear that a central computerised system with dual access by primary and secondary care, with comprehensive software would be more appropriate. This must be the future we work towards.

Reference

1   Maurois A (1989) Three Letters on the English. Taken from: *England, An Anthology* compiled by Richard Ingrams. Collins, London.

14

Case study 3: Ditching the paper in Staffordshire

Dai Evans

Context

When looking at our local journey in health informatics over the last 14 years, it is important to understand the context within which we have operated.

The old North Staffordshire Health Authority had, at its heart, the sprawling towns composing the industrial city of Stoke-on-Trent. The city had a high level of single-handed GPs among a scattering of larger practices. It is surrounded by a rural area stretching 40 miles across, from the Shropshire borders to the highest village in England at Flash, and 20 miles deep, from the Cheshire plains to the edge of Ashbourne. Small market towns, such as Leek and Cheadle, form satellite health communities with three- to four-handed practices, with remoter rural practices around the edge.

Since 1990, the primary care community has faced many organisational and workload challenges. The practices have handled the 'new contract' of the early 1990s, with its hypertension clinics, acquired new management skills with the implementation of fund-holding, endured the disbanding of health authorities and the move through primary care groups to primary care trusts. In recent times they may have switched their contractual basis to provide personal medical services or shifted into the new general medical services contract with its target-driven basis. All of these changes have had huge effects on organisational communications and 'ways of working'.

Within healthcare delivery itself, general practice has had to manage some new pressures. There has been a workload shift from secondary to primary care, compounded by more complex care pathways and higher levels of expected care. Patient expectations have changed, and they rightly demand the need to be better informed, better cared for and the right to be directly involved in decision-making. There is also an increased sense of medico-legal defensiveness, resulting in more extensive medical records. These time pressures have had to be subsumed within a falling medical workforce. Whereas a new GP post may have attracted 100 applicants in 1990, we now have several unfilled posts in the area.

Disease patterns have also shifted. Whereas we were caring for 100 diabetics in 1992, we are now caring for 260. To counter these pressures, there has been an increase in the number and role of practice nurses, alongside wider integration of primary healthcare teams. The delivery of out-of-hours care has become more rationalised with the shift from practice-based rotas to a district-wide co-operative.

Technologically we have moved from the age of the paper Lloyd-George patient record at the start of the 1990s, to the more widespread, but not universal, use of the electronic patient record, whilst communications have embraced the mobile phone, fax, internet and e-mail. The computers we use have shifted from servers with 4 mB hard drives and peripheral terminals, to today's 120 gigabyte servers running networked PCs, lap-tops and personal digital assistants. We have evolved from pure isolated 'island' systems, to all of our practices receiving electronic laboratory results, being linked to the strategic health authority demographic Exeter system, being able to make some referrals online and more recently have data extracted remotely, as in the QResearch project.

Increasingly, new staff have some basic knowledge of computers, and clinical staff often arrive with a working knowledge of general practice IT systems. In the background, the government's health informatics programmes, 'Information for Health' and more recently *Connecting for Health* (formerly the National Programme for Information Technology) have attempted to address the development of electronic working within the NHS.

The development of the electronic record over this period has become essential to surviving many of these new workload pressures and organisational initiatives. What follows is a personal view of the development of electronic ways of working, from the desktop of a North Staffordshire market town GP.

Development of e-working

At the start of the 1990s, few practices had computer systems, and those that did have them, were using them in quite limited ways. There was also a spread of different systems being used and so opportunities to learn from each other were limited. Further, the supporting health authority staff were few in number, had limited appreciation of the potential role of the computer in the consultation (as we had limited appreciation of computers) and were not therefore in a position to provide much assistance. Lastly, the system suppliers training process was aimed at a 'cascade training' of system functions, as opposed to actually how to use them for real in the consultation.

The cascade training system was fundamentally flawed for many practices for a number of reasons. First, those attending training were usually enthusiasts who would have to pass on information to reluctant colleagues. Second, they may not have been good educators in their own right and, further, they may not have been given adequate opportunity to pass on their knowledge. Carving out time in a busy practice is not always easy. Some groups of staff, such as practice nurses, may have been omitted from the cascade process and, lastly, in some cases, the staff member moved on before imparting their acquired knowledge.

Acquiring initial functional IT skills: a self-help group solution

In 1992 a small group of individuals who were using the same system came together to start sharing knowledge on how to get the best out of their computer systems. The six met monthly in a surgery, in front of a computer screen and thus founded the Three Shires User Group. Over a period of time they looked at those system functions that were essential and worked out how to best use them. They then went methodically through the remaining system functions to identify useful tips and tools. The size of the group grew by word of mouth as more practices joined. In time, the group started to extend feelers into the outside world to try and learn from other organisations such as the nascent national user groups and the Primary Health Care Specialist Group. Some of these communications involved the use of electronic bulletin boards, such as the Pry Marie Care board, to share knowledge.

We started to look at the 'management of change' and how best to implement new IT processes using needs and risk assessments, whilst learning a lot about the engagement of reluctant colleagues and staff.

Disseminating IT skills into the local community: local user groups

As the core group moved forward with its new-found expertise, others came along asking the same questions we had struggled with. Many of the group were involved in training, so it became natural to set up a series of educational workshops to disseminate our knowledge. At its peak, the meetings would attract 70–100 individuals coming from a geographical area stretching from Buxton, in north Derbyshire, across Staffordshire and Cheshire to the Welsh borders. An educational mix of small group work-shops and didactic sessions would be run in the evenings on an entirely voluntary basis. It became a useful focus for the system supplier and local health informatics staff. The success of the group probably led to other practices switching IT systems to the same supplier (and this, in turn, led to some hard lessons concerning data transfer). However, by the millennium, the core group was moving on to newer challenges and the pressures of available free time led to the slow demise of the group, although it has been partly resurrected by local health informatics staff.

Particular lessons in the development of electronic records

Over time, those developing electronic patient records had to overcome particular problems. They had to develop a structured approach to im-plementation of the records. Once demographic data was loaded onto their systems, the first job was to input repeat prescribing records by hand. Next followed the recording of audit data needed for the 'new' contract and, soon after, early use of consultation records. This was a time of experimentation in getting the best out of the systems. It was recognised that all users would need training in the development of a practice IT system. For instance, within our practice, we ensured that any locum medical staff had three training sessions before starting work, to enable them to access and input data. This made them a valuable commodity, as nearly all the practices within the area had migrated onto the same IT system. We had to identify training needs as each level of system development occurred – and meet them. It also became apparent that particular staff categories had varying exposure to training. Practice nurses, in particular, were just expected to enter data into patients' electronic records, with minimal training in the IT system and often none in the use of READ codes. This mirrors the current situation with community nursing staff.

As local users became more experienced in the use of audit, they became acutely aware of the value of data quality and this, in turn, fed the process of better data recording. It became apparent that there were three levels of IT expertise needed by users. The first was simple IT knowledge, such as using a mouse or handling Windows. The second level involved picking up the functional capabilities of the GP computer systems. This was the usual level of training provided by IT system suppliers and is akin to a car salesman pointing out where the headlight switch is and how to turn the ignition on. However, car salesmen do not instruct you how to drive, or the rules of the road, and it is this third level of actually 'how to use the system in the consultation to best effect' that users were, and still are, repeatedly asking for. There was scant support for training resources, in terms of time cost and expertise, from the NHS health informatics programme and this has probably fundamentally slowed the development of the use of IT within primary care.

Organisational impacts on training: skinning the cat another way

As the value of audit in reflecting on clinical management became apparent, other organisations helped with the training gap. The North Staffordshire Medical Audit Advisory Group (MAAG) devised a free training programme for practices in the use of GP systems' audit tools, although it was not widely taken up. The value of recording and collecting data in primary care was spotted by research workers at Keele University, and this led to the setting up of the Keele General Practice Research Network (GPRN). The fundamental hope was that if all the morbidity passing through primary care could be captured, this would be a wonderful resource for research purposes. Data quality standards were put in place and participating practices expected to meet them. Some tough lessons were learned by the Network when it was realised that the quality of data was not what it should be. There were three main reasons for this. First, we cannot hope to capture all the possible morbidity flowing though primary care. Second, there was a training gap and therefore a training programme was devised to fill the need. Third, there were some recalcitrant users, and various methods of persuasion were employed with participating practices to encourage better data recording. The programme is now in its seventh year and has demonstrated that it is possible to capture and code all patient contacts in a useful way. The training programme has borne fruit and those practices within the network stand in good stead for the rigours of data recording under the new general medical services contract. Further, the programme was adapted and used in other practices, both within the district and outside, across the country.

Keele had early links to the Collection of Healthcare Data in General Practice project (CHDGP), and its national successor, PRIMIS, has helped build a wider data quality project within the district, though still in its early days.

Regional learning networks have also had some impact in the bigger health informatics organisations, but as yet their influence is still to reach primary care, once again, perhaps for a lack of resources from central government.

Some examples of personal change management

One of the oft-repeated questions is how to persuade individuals to move forward with IT, particularly if they learned to write with pen and paper, and are nearing retirement. The reality is that it may be too difficult to engage some individuals, and the organisation may have to live with that in the short term. Learning new skills at the end of our working life may be a bridge too far. There are also issues of perceived competence and seeing a cardiac surgeon typing slowly with two fingers, into an electronic patient record, may give patients a false impression concerning their skills in the operating theatre. Attempting to concentrate on a depressed patient contemplating suicide, whilst engaging with a computer system, is not an easy task. Individuals are also often covertly afraid that they can somehow irreparably damage the whole practice IT system by their actions. This fear needs to be specifically allayed.

For each person, there has to be a positive reason to use an IT system. For most GPs, it was worth the work of hand entering repeat prescriptions onto a computer system, as it was no longer necessary to write out prescriptions by hand. But one doctor nearing retirement had taken the decision not to use the computer, for all the reasons outlined above. However, one day he noticed that when a patient arrived at the surgery to see him, the letter 'A' appeared by the patient's name on the computer screen, along with the time of arrival. This meant that if he watched the screen, he could now call the patient through to his room by tannoy, without getting up from his chair to check if the patient had arrived, leaving plenty of time to hide his cigarette. However, he had not reckoned with the screen saver, which intermittently replaced the view. He was therefore shown how to press the spacebar to bring back his desired view. This was a small key to unlock personal change for him, but subsequently he gained the confidence to press the 'L' key to mark the patient's departure, thereby alerting practice staff to his being free and available to have a cup of tea brought to him. From there, he moved on to prescribing medication using the computer, a large leap considering his early position. Interestingly, he was only able to comfortably accept this information from reception staff, not from colleagues, perhaps from fear of perceived inadequacy.

Another example from the GPRN related to an individual who was similarly nearing retirement and whose data recording was persistently not as complete as others. When he was shown audit data relating to his favourite clinical topic, he immediately wanted to know more about the disease presentation within his practice. It was pointed out to him that that information could only be gleaned if recorded, from which point he became a convert to data capture.

Process management in practice: an under-recognised requirement

It may well be that certain individuals are able to look at ways of working, or data flows, within a practice and reduce them to clear organisational pathways. But experience within North Staffordshire has shown that it is not universally employed, to the detriment of electronic record usage.

In the first example, four training practices at the forefront of IT development, agreed to carry out a joint diabetes audit to look at patient care. This was the first time the process had been undertaken in the area and among the data we looked at was the level of the last recorded glycosylated haemoglobin (HbA1) (Figure 14.1). One of the practices had not been linked to the local biochemistry laboratory for its blood test results and therefore paid someone to enter them by hand so that the data would be available within consultations. They were therefore surprised to see they had the highest level of unrecorded HbA1 results (the third column in the right-hand group). It transpired that they had not been thorough enough in their instructions. They had asked the person to enter the READ code for HbA1, but had omitted to mention that the associated blood test value should also have been entered and it subsequently was not. This state of affairs had existed for six months before we carried out our audit.

In a second example, a practice decided to summarise their patients' records onto a computer. They decided to carry it out in a systematic way, running through the patients' records alphabetically from 'A'. This they did, but did not think through the process as being part of a bigger organisational system. After a few months it was pointed out to them that they had not analysed the way information gets into electronic records, and that although

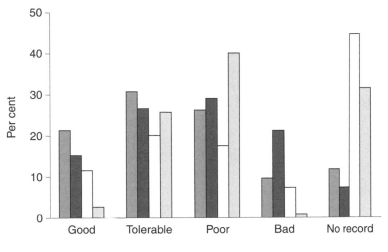

Figure 14.1 All diabetics: HbA1 records.

they were starting to handle historical data from the paper records along-side entering consultation data, a significant amount gets in from new hospital letters. This they had not accounted for and had no process in place to extract important medical information from the letters into the com-puterised patient record. Therefore all the records they had summarised over the last six months were now potentially out of date.

e-Working in the wider health community

Alongside the development of the primary care electronic record there have been other infrastructure changes that have affected communication. Some of the GP systems developed messaging programmes akin to internal e-mail. This started to provide ways of communicating electronically to members of the team and a whole new organisational concept. Previously, teams may have communicated by a number of ways, including paper in pigeon holes, telephone, message boards or carbon-copy message books. Each of these carried assumptions about whether the message would be received and acted upon. Some of the new programmes also allowed electronic task handling and forwarding, such as EMIS' 'patient notes'. This meant that we could attach a 'task' to a patient's record and forward it to a team member in the expectation that it would be actioned. This of course meant a 'business-trust' process had to be established around the ways of working.

As practices started to replace dumb terminals with PCs, this facilitated the creation of intranets with document libraries, although in reality few practices have taken advantage of this. It does mean that important documents, both internal and external, can be stored in a way that facilitates access and this has had positive advantages for e-learning, although even fewer practices have thought through the e-librarianship skills needed to develop this process (Figure 14.2).

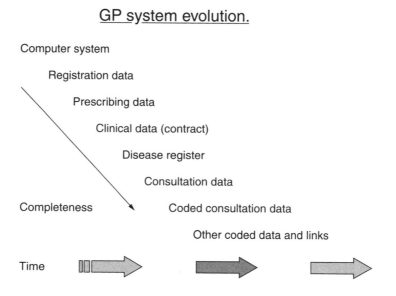

Figure 14.2 GP system evolution.

The provision of ISDN lines to practices, and subsequently district-wide e-mail facilities, has further enabled communication. We are just learning how to communicate through e-mail as a wider association of communities within the district. The cascade of drug alert information is particularly successful, as is the distribution of political (British Medical Association (BMA) and Local Medical Committee (LMC)) and other organisational information as well as other subscription services (Keele University, etc.). There are still rough edges to be sorted out though as there has not been much discussion about e-mail etiquette and we can find ourselves added automatically to e-mail distribution lists and therefore receiving e-mails of no relevance to our role. Further, there are still instances of patient-identifiable information being sent by e-mail and, in one instance, even highly sensitive information about a colleague's health status was sent to the whole district e-mail list.

As yet there are few practices engaging with patients by e-mail, as there is still work to be done on ensuring it is handled safely and securely.

Individuals are increasingly learning how to access useful information on the world wide web. Some consultations can even turn into joint learning exercises with patients on finding information about rarer diseases across the web. However, the skills to seek out reliable information, and discern good websites from poor, take some time to acquire and as yet there is no formal programme to facilitate this.

The use of computer-based records in the consultation has also provided some extra benefits for patients. It has eased communication with deaf patients who can now see their consultation (and any pertinent questions) being typed onto a screen. The provision of patient information leaflets linked to the current consultation has enhanced the education of patients concerning their medical conditions.

One particular problem concerns the 'business-trust' process around the passage of electronic patient information between organisations, and herein lies one of the major problems for the future. Over the last eight years a small number of practices have received electronic laboratory results from a nearby hospital. These have been of excellent value as they move directly into patient records after a process of patient matching and facilitate both audit and workflow in the receiving practices. However, the actual process and structure of the electronic message is not well understood by those using them. This lack of understanding led to a small free text entry being added to the message by the hospital to facilitate its internal processes. However, this entry occurred in a place where receiving systems were expecting READ-coded data. As a result, whenever the free text happened to match a READ code this code and its READ term were applied to that patient's electronic record. The receiving system handled it in such a way that the information was not immediately obvious to someone browsing the record, but it did on occasion surface. By the time we had identified it, we estimate over 1600 patients had had a code representing 'mental health disorder' added to their records across the district. In other cases, a code suggestive of cancer was added to the patient's record. Having discovered it, appropriate steps were taken to rectify the situation, but despite ensuing discussions with all the parties involved, a similar problem was repeated a few months later. This highlights the problems that may occur in the future when we are passing large amounts of electronic information between organisations.

Current position: computer-based records – successes and holes

At the start of 2004, we find ourselves in a position where all the practices in the district have computer systems. A small handful are not accredited by RFA guidelines and these are to be converted to RFA compliant systems within the year. How many practices have moved over to electronic patient records, rather than Lloyd-George records, is unclear but within Staffordshire Moorlands Primary Care Trust only two practices out of 16 have not made the move. Within the primary care trust, the average practice will have summarised its records on computer, be recording all face-to-face consultations, almost all prescriptions, be receiving electronic lab results and be scanning inbound letters with patient information.

Where are the holes in the data? Little information is recorded concerning out-of-hours patient contact as this information is received incomplete and on paper. Transcription is a job too far for some. Whilst all doctor–patient consultations may have a record, not all practice nurse contacts are recorded and only a minority of community staff contacts (health visitors, district nurses, midwives, etc.). Handling home visits is also problematic. Whilst personal data assistants and lap-top solutions are available, none of these works perfectly and so many people take paper summaries to the home to provide information and transcribe the information later onto the main system, with all the consequent problems of inaccuracy and incompleteness. Not all telephone contacts may be recorded, which may be of medico-legal significance. The prescribing records may not contain details of medication issued by other agencies, such as hospitals (for example, chemotherapy, phenylbutazone) or out-of-hours services, and may not be complete where handwritten scripts are issued, such as on home visits. The historical patient information on the computer will really only reflect that which has happened since the move to the electronic record and other subjectively important information. Increasingly, we are going to need the patient to check the validity of their own computer-based record. Some health professionals, such as optometrists, are still outside the scope of current communication. The current situation with district nurses and health visitors, alluded to above, is that they may have to record the same piece of information five times onto electronic and paper records. They get little, if any, information out of their main IT system owing to its limitations and are therefore increasingly using the GP systems.

In recent times we have just started using electronic referral systems locally. These have a long way to develop currently as it takes no information from the current clinical system. All the required information has to be re-keyed and, as it is entered into a form over the internet, the process takes at least seven minutes so is not a process that can be fitted into the limitations of a consultation. There are some electronic referral forms available that extract information from the electronic patient record, but these have to be printed out and there have been problems in getting local hospital consultants to accept their use, despite conforming to national standards.

15

Finding out more

Louise Simpson

A range of tools and resources is available to support communications and e-communications. The following is a digest of the ones we have seen and liked, and we welcome a pointer to any that you know and like (please e-mail suggestions to lou.wilson@nhs.net).

Books, papers and journals

Adair J (1997) *Effective Communication*. Pan Books, London.
Arnold E and Underman Boggs K (2003) *Interpersonal Relationships: professional communication skills for nurses*. WB Saunders, New York.
Boyce R (1997) *The Communications Revolution at Work*. SPS, London.
Kidd M (1993) Why Australian General Practitioners Don't use Computers, 7th Computer Conference of the Royal Australian College of General Practitioners, Melbourne.
Kidd MR, Connoley GL, Cesnick B and McPhee W (1993) What do medical students know about computers? *Medical Journal of Australia* **158**: 283–4.
Kurtz S, Silverman J and Draper J (1998) *Teaching and Learning Communication Skills*. Radcliffe Medical Press, Abingdon.
Littlejohn SW (2004) *Theories of Human Communication* (8e). Wadsworth Press, London.
Lloyd M and Bor R (2002) *Communication Skills for Medicine*. Churchill Livingstone, London.
Scottish Executive (2003) *Talking Matters: Developing the communication skills of doctors*. Scottish Executive, Edinburgh.

Web and CD-ROM resources

Butcher R, *The Computer in the Consultation* (www.skillscascade.com/specifics/computer_in_the_consultation.htm).

Change Management, lots of PDF files and other online resources relating to research and practical guidance about change management in the health service (www.sdo. lshtm.ac.uk/changemanagement.htm). Topics include relationships, organisational transformation and leadership through change.

Communication skills for primary care, University of Glasgow Section of General Practice and Primary Care (www.gla.ac.uk/departments/generalpractice/cpd_comm_skills.htm).

Implementing NPfIT in London (nww.imt4london.nhs.uk/londonict.htm).

Information in General Practice, a resource pack available online from five Leeds primary care trust team, developed by Karen Johnson (www.leeds.nhs.uk/iigp/).

Kidd M, *IT Linking General Practice, Hospital and Community: new roles, new rules and new challenges* (www.archi.net.au/content/index.phtml/itemId/126344).

Midwives On Line, a resource pack aimed at supporting the information needs of midwives (www.midwivesonline.com). Includes evidence, guidelines, conferences news and a chat space for healthcare professionals and parents.

Simple tips for better people-relations, from the Reputation consultancy (www.e-reputation.co.uk).

Take the palpitations out of presentations, a guide to presenting from the Reputation consultancy (www.e-reputation.co.uk).

Organisations and their websites

Accenture (www.accenture.com).

Association of Directors of Social Services Information Management Group (www.jwsolutions.co.uk/img/MaxWeb/default.asp).

Australian College of Health Informatics (www.chi.unsw.edu.au).

Australian Resource Centre for Healthcare Innovations (www.archi.net.au).

BAMM (www.bamm.co.uk).

BMA (www.bma.org.uk).

Department of Health (www.dh.gov.uk).

The Knowledge and Innovation Network (www.ki-network.org).

The Knowledge Summit (www.knowledge-summit.com).

National Primary Care Development Team (www.npdt.org).

Northumberland, Tyne and Wear Strategic Health Authority (www.ntwha.nhs.uk).

UK Council for Health Informatics Professionals (UKCHIP) (www.ukchip.org) was launched by Lord Hunt in 2004 having been formed in 2002 to promote professionalism in health informatics. It operates a voluntary register of health informatics professionals who agree to work to clearly defined standards. The website has more information about the council and a place to apply online to register as a health informatics professional.

Primary Healthcare Specialist Group of the British Computing Society (www. phcsg.org.uk).

Institute of Public Relations (www.ipr.org.uk).

Reputation (www.e-reputation.co.uk).

Communications Skills (www.comms-skills.co.uk).

Connecting for Health (www.cfh.nhs.uk).

Other materials: some useful addresses

- Department of Health, Richmond House, 79 Whitehall, London SW1A 2NL (Tel 020 7210 3000; web www.doh.gov.uk).
- General Medical Council External Relations Office, General Medical Council, 178 Great Portland Street, London W1N 6JE (Tel 020 7915 3507; web www.gmc-uk.org).
- Royal College of General Practitioners (RCGP), 14 Princes Gate, London SW7 1PM (Tel 020 7581 3232; web www.rcgp.org.uk).

16

Glossary of abbreviations

ACAS	Advisory, Conciliation and Arbitration Service
A&E	Accident & Emergency
AHC	Association of Healthcare Communicators
BAMM	British Association of Medical Managers
BMA	British Medical Association
BNF	British National Formulary
CME	Continuing medical education
CPD	Continuing professional development
DoH	Department of Health
FTE	Full-time equivalent
GMC	General Medical Council
GMS	General medical services
GP	General (medical) practitioner
GPRN	General Practice Research Network
HA	Health authority
HARP	The Health for Asylum Seekers and Refugee Portal
HimP	Health improvement programme
HORUS	Holding, obtaining, recording, using and sharing
HR	Human Resources
HRM	Human resource management
iiCR	Information in the consulting room
IPR	Individual performance review
IRS	Industrial Relations Service
IT	Information technology
LASA	London Advice Services Alliance
LMC	Local Medical Committee

LSP	Local service provider
MAAG	Medical Audit Advisory Group
MEHA	Minority Ethnic Health Awareness
MINOPS	Medicines Information Needs for Older People with Sight Loss
NCRS	NHS Care Records Service
NHS	National Health Service
NPfIT	National Programme for Information Technology
NSF	National Service Framework
PCIP	Primary Care Investment Plan
PCO	Primary care organisation
PCT	Primary care trust
PDP	Personal Development Plan
PMS	Personal medical services
PPDP	Professional Practice Development Plan
RCGP	Royal College of General Practitioners
RFA	Requirements for accreditation
RNIB	Royal National Institute for the Blind
ScHARR	School of Health and Related Research
SHA	Strategic Health Authority

Index

Page numbers in italics refer to figures or tables.

access
  environmental 99–100
  patient e-records 43–4
Accident & Emergency e-communications
      101–9
  between individuals 103
  interdepartmental 103–6
accountability issues 43–4
Als, AB 31, 33
answerphones 107
Association of Healthcare
      Communicators 4
Attenborough, David 13
'audiences' 69–74
  characteristics 70
  getting feedback 71–2
  literacy levels 56, 74
  visualising 72–4
audit
  and coding 114
  and information governance
      frameworks 51
automatic responses, and expertise
      21–2

back-up systems 109
Baker, SI 14
Blackberry use 79–80
  case studies 68–9
  instead of talking 78, 80
  see also e-mail
blind carbon copying (bcc) 69, 91–2

British Medical Association (BMA), on
      communication skills 6–7
British National Formulary (BNF) 33–4

Caldicott Guardians 50
carbon copying 91
Caroll, Lewis 79
'Cartesian theatre' 16
cascade training systems 112
central data 'spine' 7, 10
CHDGP (Collection of Healthcare Data in
      General Practice) project 115
clinical coding *see* coding
clinical guidance and e-communication
      42–3
coding 44
  errors 116–17, 119
  guidance sources 42
  training issues 42, 113–14
communication
  boundaries and range 12–13
  models 13–15, *14–15*
  principles 15
communication in the NHS
  background 6–7
  current policy initiatives 7–8
  delivering key messages 75
  diagnosing problem issues 61–4
  evaluating approaches 77
  information sources 122–4
  and meaningfulness 62–3
  patient perspectives 8–9, 72–3

teamworking skill requirements 40–2
understanding context issues 76–7
see also e-mail; interdisciplinary
teamwork
Communication Skills Education for Doctors
(BMA 2003) 6–7
Communities of Practice (Wenger) 20
computers in consultations 26–34, 108–9
aims of use 33–4
confidentiality issues 32
effect on patients 29–30, 33
knowledge flow 27–9, *28*
knowledge models (Robinson and
Heywood) 27, *28*
practical tips 31–2
confidentiality
computer use in consultations 32
photocopying and facsimile 108
and privacy 104
and security 49
telecommunications 107
written communications 106
Connecting for Health (DoH 2000) 7–8, 111
consciousness 15–17
consent *see* patient consent
consultations
knowledge flow 27–9, *28*
knowledge use models (Robinson and
Heywood) 27, *27*
using computers 29–34, 108–9
see also GP surgeries
Crisp, Nigel 4
cross boundary care 10, 103–6
e-communication 43–4

Dance, FEX 14, *15*
Darwin, Charles 13
data coding *see* coding
data spine *see* central data 'spine'
decision-making
doctor-patient 9
and 'group-think' 38–41
interdisciplinary 37–8
delegation 41
Delivering 21st Century IT for the NHS
(DoH 2002) 7–8
Dennett, DC 16
Descartes, René 16
digital images 107
disability, access to healthcare 99–100

discharge information 108–9
diversity issues 53–6
case studies (MINOPS project)
97–100
electronic language assistance 56–8
information needs 54–6
documentation
face-to-face meetings 105–6
telephone conversations 107, 120
transcription issues 120
Domasio, A 17
Douglas, Colin 29
drugs
information sources 33–4
see also prescribing electronically
Dylan, Bob 12

e-communication
background 6–7
current policy initiatives 7–8
delivering key messages 75
developing policies 87–9, 91–2
diagnosing problem issues 61–4
evaluating approaches 77
information sources 122–4
and meaningfulness 62–3
patient perspectives 8–9, 72–3
teamworking skill requirements 40–2
understanding context issues 76–7
see also e-mail; interdisciplinary
teamwork
e-communication devices *see* Blackberry
use; e-mail
e-communication policies
development considerations 87–9
specific issues 91–2
e-communities, GP-UK 42
e-mail
developing policy protocols 87–9
focusing on key messages 85–7
influence of sender reputation 81–3
making content effective 84–7
message checking 45
mistakes and indiscretions 44, 67, 86,
92–3
risk management 80, 87–9, 92–4
trust issues 45, 69
unintended consequences 67–9
use of blind carbon copying (bcc) 69,
91–2

use of carbon copying 91
use of 'forwarding' exchanges 92
volume overload 43, 68
when to send 88
writing headers 83–4
see also Blackberry use; interdisciplinary
    teamwork
Electronic Health Horizons (NHS Executive
    2000) 55
electronic portable data assistants *see*
    Blackberry use
emotion, psychological basis 17
errors *see* mistakes
ethnic minorities
    case studies (MINOPS project) 97–100
    language difficulties 53–6
    technology assistance 56–8
evaluating e-communication strategies 77
evidence-based guidance, access 9–10
experts, and knowledge flows 27–9
*The Expression of Emotions in Man and
    Animals* (Darwin) 13

face-to-face meetings 41–2
    documentation difficulties 105–6
    language problems 105
faxed information 108
feedback, 'reputation' audits 64, 71–2
Follett, MP 38
forwarding e-mails 92
Freedom of Information Act 67

general practice, and information
    governance 50–1
General Practice Research Network
    (GPRN) 114
geographic boundary issues *see* cross
    boundary care
*Good Practice Guidelines for General Practice
    Electronic Patient Records*
    (GPC–RCGP) 50–1
Gower Handbook of Internal Communication
    (Newbold and Scholes) 40–1
GP surgeries
    accommodating disabilities 98–100
    case study of IT systems 117–19, *118*
    see also consultations
GP-UK e-community 42
GPRN (General Practice Research
    Network) 114

Greatbach, D *et al.* 30
'group-think' problems 38–9
    prevention tips (Janis) 39
Guide to the internet: electronic mail
    (Pallen) 80

handheld e-communication devices *see*
    Blackberry use
handwriting, and legibility 108
HARP (Health for Asylum Seekers and
    Refugees Portal) 57
Hawthorne, K 56
headers 83–4
Health for Asylum Seekers and Refugees
    Portal (HARP) 57
health inequalities, and ethnic
    minorities 56–7
helix model of communication 14, *15*
HORUS (Holding, obtaining, recording,
    using and sharing) framework
    47, *48*
The Houseman's Tale (Douglas) 29

iiCR (Information in the consulting room)
    project 30–1
informatics model of communication
    (Shannon) 13–14, *14*
Information in the consulting room *see* iiCR
    (Information in the consulting
    room) project
information delivery
    audience characteristics 70
    audience literacy 56, 74
    language diversity issues 53–8
information governance 47–51
    definitions 47
    general importance 10, 49
    and HORUS framework 47, *48*
    in general practice 50–1
    in primary care 49–50
    national aims 49
    and security 49
    toolkits and guidelines 49–51
    as trust framework 10
    'workstreams' and coding 44
information leaflets, and ethnic language
    issues 56–7
information sharing, guidelines 50
information sources on e-communication
    122–4

informed consent 105
  guidelines 50
integrated care records service *see* NHS Care
  Records Service
interdisciplinary communication
  case studies 103–6, 117–9
  face-to-face 41–2, 105
  photocopying and facsimile 108
  required skills 40–1
  telecommunications 107
  written 106
interdisciplinary teamwork 10
  communication skills 40–1
  decision-making 37–8
  'group-think' problems 38–9
  issues around e-communication 42–5
interpreters 55, 98
intrapersonal communication 12–13
  and consciousness 15–19, *18–19*
ISDN lines 118

Janis, Irving 39
jargon 20, 66
joint learning 119

Keele University, General Practice Research
  Network (GPRN) 114–15
Kidd, Prof. Michael 10
knowledge flows
  in consultations 27–9, *28*
  models (Robinson and Heywood) 27, *28*
  new guidance 42–3
language 13
  case studies (MINOPS project) 97–100
  diversity issues 53–8
  for e-mail communication 71
LASA (London Advice Services Alliance)
  multikulti project 57
Life of Mammals (Attenborough) 13
listening skills and ecommunication
  41
literacy 56, 74
Littlejohn, Stephen 38
London Advice Services Alliance (LASA)
  multikulti project 57
Lothian University Hospitals NHS Trust
  8–9

Man Watching (Morris) 13
managing e-risk 80, 87–9, 92–4

Maurois, André 101
meaning, and jargon 20
medication lists 107
Medicines Information Needs for Older
  People with Sight Loss (MINOPS)
  project 97–100
meetings
  face-to-face 41–2
  misuse of e-mail 78, 80
MEHA (Minority Ethnic Health Awareness)
  Project UK 57
memory 17–18
  and consciousness 17–19
  and narrative 19–20
messages
  delivering key points 75
  writing e-mails 85–7
  see also e-mail
middle management 43
MINOPS *see* Medicines Information needs
  for Older people with Sight Loss
  project
Minority Ethnic Health Awareness (MEHA)
  Project UK 57
mistakes
  answerphone messages 107
  assessing risk 93–4
  e-mail use 44, 67, 86, 92–3
  inputting codes 116–17, 119
  lost patient records 106
  photocopying and facsimile 108
mobile phones, and digital images
  107
Morris, Desmond 13
motivation to learn 115–16
mypil.com website 56

The Naked Ape (Morris) 13
narrative 19–20
National Programme for IT (NPfIT) *see*
  Connecting for Health (DoH 2000)
networking and ecommunication
  42
New South Wales Multicultural Health
  Communication Service 57
Newbold, A and Scholes, E 40–1
NHS Care Records Service 7–8, 10
  see also patient records
NHS Direct, on multilingual information
  initiatives 57

NHS Information Authority, on information
    governance 51
The NHS Plan (DoH 2000) 7–8
    and information governance 49
non-verbal communication 13, 20–1
North Staffordshire Health Authority
    e-communication initiatives
        110–21
    context 110–11
    disseminating skills 112, 113–14
    early developments 112
    electronic records initiatives 11304
    personal change stories 115–16
    process management issues 116–17
    training considerations 114–16
    wider community contexts 117–19

'off-road' coding 42
organisations
    as communication barrier 6–7
    structural changes 43
Our Healthier Nation (DoH 1998) 55
outcomes in e-communication 67–9

Pallen, Mark 80
patient consent 105
    guidelines 50
patient information needs
    case studies (MINOPS project) 97–100
    language issues 53–8
patient medication lists 107
patient records
    access during consultations 33
    access guidelines 50
    confidentiality issues 104, 106, 108
    drawings and diagrams 109
    historical data 120
    recording communication needs 98–9
    security considerations 106, 107, 109
    transcription issues 120
    verification issues 120
    see also NHS Care Records Service
patient satisfaction
    with doctor-patient communication 8–9
    with NHS 4
peer opinions 64
photocopying and facsimile 108
Plato's cave 18–19, *19*
portable e-communication devices *see*
        Blackberry use

practice nurses
    documenting patient contacts 120
    role changes 111
    prescribing electronically 29–30, 32, 115
    information sources 33–4
PRIMIS 115
    on data quality education 42
privacy, and confidentiality 104
PRODIGY 29
Pry Marie Care board 112
psychological model of communication
    (Baker) 14

QResearch project 111

READ codes 113, 116–17
    see also coding
referral pathways 120–1
    A & E–primary care 108–9, 10405
repeat prescribing 115
report writing and e-communication 42
reputation audits 64
    and general feedback 71–2
RFA guidelines 120
Riccardi, VM and Kurtz, SM 15
risk management, e-mail use 80, 87–9,
        92–4
Robinson, PJ and Heywood, P 27, *27*

Samuels, Paul 43
satisfaction surveys *see* patient satisfaction
security issues
    computer use 108–9
    and information governance 49
    see also mistakes
Shannon informatics model 13–14, *14*
sharing information *see* information sharing
Shifting the Balance of Power (DoH 2002) 4
social conditioning, use of jargon 20
Sowerby Centre 30, 34
stories and narrative 19–20
strategies for e-communication 65–78
    basic considerations 65–6
    defining aims 67–9
    delivering key messages 75
    evaluating approaches 77
    identifying appropriate channels 74
    identifying audience characteristics
        69–74
    understanding contexts 76

stress, from e-communication overload
43, 68
subliminal communication 20–1
symbols 13

teamwork *see* interdisciplinary teamwork
'technophobes' 44
telecommunications 107
documentation issues 120
Theories of Human Communication
(Littlejohn) 38
Three Shires User Group 112
training
cascade systems 112
on consultations and computer use
30–1, 34
different levels 114
and motivation to learn
115–16
transcription issues 120
translation services 55–6
technology assistance 56–7

trust 3–4, 10
and clinical data entry 45
and e-mail use 45, 92
and group-think 38
and information governance
10

vision
and consciousness 16–17
neurology 16–17
visualisation techniques, for better
communication 72–4

web-based information sources
122–3
Wenger, Etienne 20
Wilson, R *et al.* 56
working memory 17–18
consciousness 17–19
and narrative 19–20
working pattern changes 3–4
written communications 106